DATE DUE

3 8 17 ILL			

Demco, Inc. 38-293

of related interest

Involving Families in Care Homes
A Relationship-Centred Approach to Dementia Care
Bob Woods, John Keady and Diane Seddon
ISBN 978 1 84310 229 8
Bradford Dementia Group Good Practice Guides

Design for Nature in Dementia Care
Garuth Chalfont
ISBN 978 1 84310 571 8
Bradford Dementia Group Good Practice Guides

The Pool Activity Level (PAL) Instrument for Occupational Profiling
A Practical Resource for Carers of People with Cognitive Impairment
Third edition
Jackie Pool
ISBN 978 1 84310 594 7
Bradford Dementia Group Good Practice Guides

Person-Centred Counselling for People with Dementia
Making Sense of Self
Danuta Lipinska
Foreword by Brian Thorne
ISBN 978 1 84310 978 5

Remembering Yesterday, Caring Today
Reminiscence in Dementia Care: A Guide to Good Practice
Pam Schweitzer and Errollyn Bruce
Foreword by Faith Gibson
ISBN 978 1 84310 649 4
Bradford Dementia Group Good Practice Guides

The Activity Year Book
A Week by Week Guide for Use in Elderly Day and Residential Care
Anni Bowden and Nancy Lewthwaite
ISBN 978 1 84310 963 1

CONNECTING THROUGH MUSIC WITH PEOPLE WITH DEMENTIA

A GUIDE FOR CAREGIVERS

Robin Rio

Jessica Kingsley Publishers
London and Philadelphia

First published in 2009
by Jessica Kingsley Publishers
116 Pentonville Road
London N1 9JB, UK
and
400 Market Street, Suite 400
Philadelphia, PA 19106, USA

www.jkp.com

Library of Congress Cataloging in Publication Data
Rio, Robin.
    Connecting through music with people with dementia : a guide for caregivers
/ Robin Rio.
        p. ; cm.
    Includes bibliographical references.
    ISBN 978-1-84310-905-1 (pb : alk. paper) 1. Dementia–Patients–Care. 2.
Music therapy for older people. 3. Caregivers. I. Title.
    [DNLM: 1. Dementia–therapy. 2. Music Therapy–methods. WM 220 R585c
2009]
    RC521.R46 2009
    616.89'1654–dc22

                                                        2008038126

British Library Cataloguing in Publication Data
A CIP catalogue record for this book is available from the British Library

ISBN 978 1 84310 905 1

Printed and bound in Great Britain by
Athenaeum Press, Gateshead, Tyne and Wear

CONTENTS

DEDICATION

This book is dedicated to my parents,
Anne and Sebastian

PREFACE

I am amazed that I have spent over ten years sharing music with older people who have cognitive losses, but I have. The truth is I have found that many people who have difficulty in day to day living because of dementia are still able to communicate, continue to be excellent company, and are avid lovers of music. But I didn't always feel this way. My first few "nursing home experiences" were actually somewhat bleak and personally distressing. I was left shaken up and not at all convinced of the power of music to provide comfort and meaningful experience, and especially unsure of my ability to make a difference in the lives of the people who most needed my help.

As a young adult, I worked as a nursing assistant in an extended-care facility. The job was extremely demanding, and I always felt a little guilty that I couldn't spend more time with each resident just talking and helping with important but "non-essential" things, like reading his mail to him or holding his hand. These are the types of activities that have more recently come to be called "quality of life," to him, essentials like bathing, feeding, dressing, and medications took priority.

Several years later, after I had finished my music therapy coursework, I was given an opportunity for volunteer work with a music therapist who was working in a nursing home. The therapist gave me a list of people to visit at bedside. They were people that she didn't have in any group sessions owing to their extreme frailty, and they were rather isolated. Most of them were unable to converse or move independently. Because the residents couldn't respond, I had no idea if my music reached them or not, and I didn't have the experience or song repertoire to know how to make a meaningful connection.

The following year I was offered a music therapy job in a nursing home with an entirely different outcome. I had a wonderful therapeutic recreation department to work in, which was a secure and educational environment for me. The director of the therapeutic recreation program knew little about music therapy, but she was kind and helpful, was a wonderful role model for how to interact with the residents, and made me feel a part of the team of care providers. I had the support of other activities workers, volunteers, and nursing staff to help me negotiate the world of the frail elderly. Most of these elderly residents had moderate to severe cognitive losses with memory impairment and a range of sensory and physical impairments. Of course, these losses were the reason they needed the help of a long-term care setting. What I came to find out after just a few weeks of consistent intervention on my part, was that when presented in a gentle and simple manner, many of these older adults were at their best—and enjoying life most—when they were involved in an interactive music experience. I had finally solved the mystery of bringing music to the person with dementia. *I needed guidance and support in implementing my music program.* It wasn't easy, and required concrete examples and lots of time with seasoned caregivers, but I now had friendly and encouraging people to share the burdens, stresses, and joys of caring for people with multiple needs and complex issues caused by Alzheimer's and related diseases. The guidance and direction I have received and learned from over the years is what I am hoping to provide for you.

INTRODUCTION

Using music to enhance interaction with a person who has dementia is a process that can be learned over time, with this book as a primary resource. Developing a sense of comfort with making sounds and singing, playing rhythms on percussion, and using recorded music effectively can be achieved by any caregiver who is interested in bringing a more rich and meaningful experience to a person who suffers from memory loss.

This book explores simple techniques to develop ability in singing and "sounding" in the caregiver, which may then be shared with the person who is receiving the music. Because a person with more advanced dementia may no longer be as self-conscious as he once was, it is generally the caregiver who needs to become "desensitized" to any anxieties or embarrassment associated with singing or making musical noises that will be heard by others. As in any learning process, the more positive experiences a person has, the more confident and capable he or she will become. As we become more capable, our natural abilities are brought forth, and sharing our musical experiences with others becomes comfortable and easy to do. This book is intended to be used as an interactive tool in creating a musical atmosphere for time shared with someone who has dementia. The caregiver may begin immediately, at whatever level of ability he or she has, by moving and singing along with recorded music. The caregiver can then gradually provide more music from his or her own voice and percussive accompaniment, and use the recorded music only as needed. The best and most meaningful music that can be shared between a caregiver and the person she is caring for is that which is produced in the moment, between the two people who are interacting together. The familiar sound and flexibility of the "live" voice of a familiar person is often preferred over a recording. The benefits of singing and moving to music can be appreciated and enjoyed by the caregiver as well as the person who has dementia.

Sally sits in her wheelchair outside the door to her bedroom, cuddling a small doll. As is normal for her, she seems lost in her own world. When I come up to her, she starts and looks up in confusion, even though we'd sung together just a few days before. She mumbles incoherently now. Looking into her perfect blue eyes, I say, "Hi, Sally, my name is Robin. May I sing with you?" I sing, "Tumbalalaika," a lovely Yiddish song with a rocking, lullaby quality that seems to match her mood. After a few repetitions, she begins to smile and nod her head to the music. When the song ends, I ask if I may hold her baby doll so that she can hold one of my instruments to play along. "Shh—" she says, resisting my suggestion, and clasping her baby doll even more tightly. She looks at the doll lovingly. I begin to sing, "Oh, You Beautiful Doll," which acknowledges her and what she is doing, and the rhythm of the music gradually brings the energy level a little higher. Next, I sing, "You Must Have Been a Beautiful Baby," remembering that she has shuffled her feet in a kind of sitting dance to this standard tune on an earlier visit. As before, Sally moves her feet in time to the music as I sing and play guitar. I put a tambourine under her foot, and she hears herself jingle with each beat. We are making music together, and Sally is smiling. She looks comfortable and relaxed, and no longer appears confused or preoccupied with the doll she is holding. She is "in the moment" with me, living in the present, interacting socially with me like an old friend would.

Years of music therapy work with people who suffered from dementia, training interns, and university teaching eventually led me to a wonderful project conducted at a nursing home in New York. I was asked, as part of a larger program, to help family members and nursing assistants who cared for residents with advanced dementia to learn how to incorporate music into their regular routine of care. The residents who qualified to participate in the project were unable to care for most, if any, of their daily living needs: they needed help feeding themselves, changing clothes, going to the bathroom, and so on. These residents were also unable to communicate their most basic thoughts and feelings effectively. The caregivers had no special training in music or therapy prior to this project. My goal for caregivers was to enable them to use music to improve the quality of interactions with residents suffering from dementia, by learning simple musical techniques that could help them to achieve moments of genuine connection.

I have outlined the steps that you, the caregiver, may take to communicate in a more meaningful way with the individual or individuals in your life who suffer from dementia. No doubt, dementia presents some significant challenges in the area of communication. But it's worth attempting because, in a surprising number of cases, even when a confused person has difficulty communicating via conversation and has stopped behaving in the "typical" way, she or he may still be able to engage in meaningful interpersonal interactions using music, various sounds, gestures, expressions, and movement. I've seen both subtle and startling breakthroughs countless times. Following the steps I detail here, you can better relate to the person or people in your life who seem to have lost many social and intellectual capabilities. To succeed, you need only have an open mind and a willingness to share music with the person in need of care.

Here are the main things you will learn from this self-study book.

- You will find out if there is any music that is particularly meaningful to the resident, with the help of anyone who has known the person with dementia for a long time or who knows her or his preferences.

- You will listen to recordings of music that was

popular when the person with dementia was a young adult.

- You will sing along with recordings of music you believe your resident will know and enjoy hearing.

- You will borrow or buy a small variety of percussion instruments and a CD player, iPod®, or any other way to play recordings.

- You will meet with the resident as often as is comfortable—any amount is helpful, and short frequent visits are best.

- You will begin by leading the resident in singing, playing a simple rhythm, or just exploring sound on a percussion instrument, and moving to music (while providing the resident with appropriate physical support as needed).

- You will carefully observe the resident's responses to music, noticing eye contact, facial expressions, gestures, body movement, words, and sounds.

- You will become familiar with percussion instruments by playing them without accompaniment and along with recorded or live music, both for and with the resident.

- You will use music that seems the most familiar and has elicited the best response in your visits at the beginning of the visit to initiate comfort and closeness, and at the end to help ease the transition of ending the music session and providing closure.

- Based on the resident's interests and abilities, songs are learned and added, and favorites are continued.

If this sounds like a lot, take heart. All of those who completed a learning experience similar to that outlined above were able to successfully apply the techniques they learned, often in fewer than six weeks after two training sessions per week. If you are not able to have a music therapist available for consultation, you might wonder about whether you'll be able to do all of this. Just think of this book as my way of assisting you through the steps needed to learn and share music. Of course, a live person is an asset, but if you are interacting through music without the guidance of a consulting music therapist, this book is the next best thing. Feel free to use these music exercises and songs throughout the day, as often as you like, knowing that you really can use music very informally and frequently, as long as you and the resident seem to enjoy it.

In some instances, the person with dementia may not respond to music. This may be discouraging, but it does not mean you have failed in learning to apply music. Since we are never certain what another person actually hears, it is well worth the effort to try to use music for interaction in hopes that some of the sounds are reaching the individual with advanced dementia, even when he is unable to show us with an obvious response. The only time you will want to stop using music is if you notice that your resident isn't enjoying it. You may take a break and try again later.

I've repeated and expanded on many of the music practices and techniques that I have outlined above for in-service training and presentations developed for nursing staff, family caregivers, activity directors, and for the education of music therapy interns and fieldwork students, and this book is the result. You may find it helpful to enlist the support of music and activities professionals as you are learning, and for follow up. Sometimes just visiting and observing a music therapist, social worker, activities or therapeutic recreation professional can make a world of difference. You may even hire someone to help you get started and give you advice at the beginning and periodically as you continue. There is a Resources section in the Appendix that can provide some places to look for assistance. I believe that anyone who has a love of music and a desire to help can develop musical connections for better communication and more meaningful interaction with those suffering from dementia.

The suggestions and ideas in the following chapters are meant to be added to whatever information you may already have. If you are currently a caregiver, you know your resident in a special way that no one else does. If the person in need of care is a relative or friend, you probably have memories of this person when he or she was a thriving, competent, and vital individual. Those past experiences are quite valuable in determining the musical interests of a person who may no longer be able to give you information directly. Sometimes, the person with Alzheimer's disease or some other form of dementia may actually have a shift in personality that makes them seem unfamiliar to those who know them. He may be more accepting of different styles of music at this stage in his life than before he experienced cognitive changes. It can be helpful to have both knowledge of the resident prior to illness and insight into his present-day interests and reactions to music. If you are a professional caregiver, such as a nursing assistant, nurse, or activities worker, or are a volunteer, it is likely that you also have a very special and unique relationship with your resident(s). With music you can learn new ways of enriching your experiences with the person who suffers from dementia.

Using music as a form of expanding your possibilities of expression and communication relies heavily on your ability to establish a sense of trust with the resident. It is truly amazing how quickly this rapport may be established when efforts are applied systematically, frequently, and with an enthusiastic and caring attitude. It is not the quality of the music presented, or the proficiency of the person presenting the music, that makes the most difference. It is the willingness to use sound in a variety of ways that can have a positive effect on the relationship with your resident.

1

ALL YOU NEED TO KNOW ABOUT MUSIC

Maybe you have never played a musical instrument, or perhaps the only singing you do is in the shower. On the other end of the musical spectrum, perhaps you have been listening to symphonies all your life and always took the lead in your high school musicals, but have little idea on how to transfer your love of music into a communication tool for a person who has cognitive challenges. Although this book was created for caregivers of dementia residents in a nursing home environment (and for this reason "resident" is used for the most part in place of "loved one" or "person with dementia" or "the person with cognitive challenges"), it is still relevant for anyone who is interested in learning more about using music therapeutically. Music therapy students and therapists who are working with the geriatric population for the first time may benefit from the information offered. Experienced therapists who are interested in training volunteers or staff in a clinical or home-bound setting will also find this book helpful. Those who want to become more involved in improving the quality of life of someone who may be suffering from a different type of disability, such as a traumatic brain injury or a stroke, could adapt the suggestions offered here as needed. Whatever your background, almost everyone has some experience with making music, listening to music, or moving to music, and I'm going to help you to expand on these positive experiences.

Here's a true story. I heard strains of "Let Me Call You Sweetheart" as I walked into the large dining room in the nursing home where the entertainment was to be held, expecting to see the "one-man band" that was scheduled to perform. Instead, I saw the recreation director, a wonderful woman who happened to be deaf. She wore two hearing aids and was an excellent lip-reader (also called a "speech reader"). She was leading a sing-along to fill in the time while waiting for the one-man band. She was not able to match pitch very well owing to her profound hearing loss, but she was a natural, enthusiastic leader with a great attitude and generous spirit. The residents loved her, and no one seemed to notice or to mind that she wasn't singing in tune or with completely accurate rhythm. The residents and visitors happily sang along with the familiar songs, and there wasn't even any accompaniment! Remember this story. And, especially, remember that it's not the level of musicianship or the quality of your voice that makes for the most meaningful interactions. It's a sense of fun and engagement. Truly, a willing heart and a short, simple repertoire of well-known songs are all that are needed to begin music sessions with your loved one.

So, without being perfectionists, we will take a look at the main elements of music, and what you need to do to bring enjoyable music to others. The most prominent elements are melody and rhythm, with a little bit of harmony included for those who have a musical background. Add in your own unique sound, which is the color in music, and then add some dynamics—the fast, slow, loud, and soft of it—and you are on your way!

Melody is the tune—the part you can hum or sing along with. Harmony occurs when more than one note is played or sung at the same time. Harmony may be played, on an instrument like a guitar or piano, or provided by another voice or voices. The rhythm is what you tap your toes to—the way the beats are organized. We are aware of music from our earliest recollection, and musicality provides functional communication from birth (Darnley-Smith and Patey 2003) through sounds indicating needs and desires that the parent is able to interpret and respond to. Because music and sound are used communicatively from very early on, before words and language have developed, it only makes sense that the same use of human's innate musicality will carry on after a person's ability to verbalize has diminished.

MELODY

A melody may be simple or complex. It may be easy to sing and remember, or very difficult. One of the most striking, timeless melodies is "Over the Rainbow." It is not necessarily easy to sing, but very easy to recognize because of its melody. The big jump up at the very beginning, in the first word "some-where," makes the song unique from the start. In recent years, with the evolution of popular music and rap, melody has taken less importance and rhythm is often the driving force. But for most of the people who are suffering from memory loss caused by dementia from Alzheimer's or related diseases, melody is still very important.

Melody and harmony belong to the same key, which can be major or minor. We usually think of music in a major key as sounding happy, and a minor key as sad or sentimental, although there are exceptions to this rule. The key also influences how high or how low in pitch the melody will be. The majority of popular American music is in a major key, as well as many traditional and celebration songs like "Jingle Bells" and "Happy Birthday." Examples of songs in minor keys are the "Anniversary Waltz" and the jazz standard, "Autumn Leaves."

Yiddish, Israeli and traditional Jewish heritage music, and Middle Eastern music are frequently in minor keys, as is a variety of classical music, art songs, and folk music of various cultures. These songs are not considered sad, even though they are in a minor key, because they represent cultures whose relationship with music relies on different sound combinations than the associations many Americans have with music. This reminds us once again of the importance of providing music that is specific to the individual, based on her culture, personal style, and family history, as much as possible.

I am third-generation Italian on my father's side of the family. My grandparents emigrated to the USA in the early 1900s, with many of their countryfolk from southern Italy, coming through Ellis Island in New York. My grandfather was very proud of his work ethic, and told us how he applied his craft of haircutting while on the long ocean voyage, trimming the hair of other passengers to earn what he could. (An Italian barber—what could be more traditional than that!) My grandmother, Nonna, told us stories of her younger days in Siracusa, Sicily, where she was a·teacher in a private girls' school. They settled in Boston and did their best to assimilate into the American culture while maintaining some of the customs and traditions of their native land. They made delicious Italian meals and sang the popular and folk songs of their youth, with Grandpa accompanying on his mandolin. In her later years, Nonna began losing her memory. Grandpa did everything he could to keep her active and well-fed, even when she started refusing food. He made her a concoction of an Ensure® shake and Kalhúa because that was the only way she would take any calories. The "spoonful of sugar" (with a little alcohol thrown in) seemed to work and Nonna remained social, despite her memory loss. Instead of saying she no longer recognized us, she'd say, "Do I know you? I haven't seen you in so long! Where have you been?" with a playful grin and a twinkle in her eye, teasing. As the disease progressed further, she began speaking solely in Italian, and my Grandpa would translate. Her favorite song from her youth remained a favorite long after she was able to recognize me, her granddaughter. I sang "Santa Lucia" to her in Italian when I visited, and she always smiled in recognition. By the end of the first refrain she would join in, singing the words to the timeless melody.

This next list offers suggestions on how to work with a melody using some simple and fun changes to how you would ordinarily sing a song. Since so many popular songs are rather short, you will want to repeat songs at least a few times until your resident has a chance to really hear and mentally process what you are doing. Try some of the following suggestions each time you sing a song to add more variety and personal touch to your repertoire.

TEN WAYS TO MAKE A MELODIC CONNECTION

1. Hum the tune gently, warming your voice.

2. Sing the tune with the words, lightly and not too fast.

3. Sing it as softly as you can, almost a whisper, but with intensity.

4. Sing the tune on your favorite syllable (*la-la, doo-doo*, etc.).

5. Sing the song like an opera singer.

6. Sing the melody up-tempo, like a march or dance tune.

7. Rap the lyrics with no tune at all, or recite them as a poem.

8. Try the words to a different tune, for example "Jingle Bells" to the tune of "Silent Night."

9. Imitate the sound and motions of a trumpet "toot toot" or harp "plink plink," etc.

10. Try singing like your favorite musical artist.

RHYTHM

Rhythm can be broken down into two main categories: double meter and triple meter. When the pulse is in four beats, it is referred to as 4/4 time. The basic beat may be counted: 1–2–3–4, 1–2–3–4, etc. The bulk of music we listen to in the USA and western European countries is written in 4/4 time, and can be heard in swing tunes, 50s rock, current contemporary pop, rap, tango...the list goes on. Triple meter can be classified most often as 3/4 time, which is the beat used in a waltz. In 3/4 time, the count is 1–2–3, 1–2–3, etc. Many of the older popular songs use this, for example "Let Me Call You Sweetheart" and "When Irish Eyes Are Smiling." "Amazing Grace" and "Silent Night" are examples of traditional or religious music that uses 3/4 time. "Rock-a-bye Baby" and other lullabies also use 3/4 time. Ethnic music which incorporates the use of 3/4 time may be found in "Too-ra-loo-ra-loo-ral," "Cielito Lindo," and "Arirang."

Drum circles are an ancient mode of music-making that has gained a remarkable resurgence in popularity in a new generation of music-makers. Just as our parents and grandparents enjoyed making music by singing songs accompanied by piano or stringed instruments, people are now enjoying participation in drum circles as a way of being actively engaged in music-making. It is a way for modern people to participate in making music without formal training, and in community with others.

Although we often associate drumming with the male rock drummer, women were some of the earliest carriers of rhythm. Women carrying drums are depicted in the art of many cultures throughout the Mediterranean and the Middle East, beginning as early as 900 BC (Redmond 1997). Women were drumming to enhance their spiritual life, to connect with nature, and to communicate with each other. Drumming was done as a ritual and for developing a sense of belonging and unity.

Fast-forward to the 1920s: the "trap set" had developed out of the New Orleans jazz and blues movement percussion "contraption" that added elements of drum and percussion instruments from all over the world, including snare and bass drum from Europe, cymbals from Turkey, cowbells, woodblocks, and gongs, all from their respective parts of the world (Hart 1990). Latin, Native American, African, and Indian musical cultures have all influenced our sense of modern rhythm and added to the wonderful array of instruments available to us today.

In a recent workshop with caregivers of people who have a loved one with dementia, I provided hand drums and shakers of various sizes and shapes to the group of approximately 25 people who were in the age range 35–75. None of them had been to a drum circle before, and none had any previous training in music, at least none that any of them would admit to. We warmed up by doing breathing and vocal exercises that are outlined in an upcoming chapter. Next, we hummed and then sang a familiar song together, and then played rhythms together on our drums and shakers. Everyone was able to participate in the music-making, and the group became quite animated and energetic. We drummed for about 15 minutes, and I asked the group members to share their comments. "That was so much fun!" "That was really relaxing!" "I didn't feel self-conscious, even though I never tried this before." "When I got off (the beat), I could just look at someone else to get back on. I didn't have to worry about singing on pitch or what the words were." "The time went really fast."

In modern society it seems we may be lacking in knowing how to connect with other people in creative ways. Drumming can fill a need for community-building and meaningful interaction in our fast-paced lives. It is also a way to "give back" or restore ourselves when we are under stress. During participation in group drumming, rhythmic entrainment develops and helps us to feel connected and unified. This entrainment is the way that we naturally beat in synchrony with each other, and is a process that enhances our sense of group experience (Bittman et al. 2003). This assimilating to the beat is something that usually happens without effort. It is actually harder to play against the rhythm of others than it is to play along with the beat. Rhythm can stimulate movement in the body. It can produce reactions as subtle as a finger-moving or a toe-wiggling, to obvious motions such as clapping, dancing, or beating a tambourine.

PERCUSSION INSTRUMENTS

Rhythms can be played on a variety of percussion instruments to accompany singing and recorded music. These percussion instruments may also be played unaccompanied. One effective technique is for both resident and care giver to explore the instrument together. Consider it an introduction to the instrument. Just make different sounds and don't be concerned about playing a specific song. You may have to introduce the same instrument each time you are together, and that's perfectly okay—in fact, it's a great way to begin a music visit because it makes for a good review. When purchasing instruments, try them out in the store. You should like the quality of the sound produced by the instrument as well as its appearance. Be sure the instrument is safe, with no sharp edges. Take into consideration the weight of the instrument and the dexterity needed to play it. Finally, remember the capabilities of the people who will be playing it.

The following are suggested percussion instruments. They can be used to help establish rhythm, to play along with recorded music or live singing, or for exploration of sounds. They can also be used to play expressively what you feel like playing, with no particular set of musical rules. Playing percussion instruments together with visitors or other residents can be a nice way to bring people together, as long as efforts are made not to become too loud for those with sensitivities to sound. The acoustics of the space should also be taken into consideration. If a room has too many hard surfaces, the sound may become muddled when the noises reverberate, which can make for an unpleasant sound environment and possible overstimulation.

Shakers come in many shapes and sizes, the most common being of Latin origin and called the "maraca." Most cultures have some form of shaker, and they are easy to hold and manipulate. Some maracas, like those sold in souvenir shops, are decorative in nature and not really meant to be played. Be sure that your maraca or shaker is well-made and intended for an adult. It is important to use instruments that are appropriate for adults, but easy to use. There are many children's instruments that are plastic and inexpensive, and unfortunately may have a poor sound quality. Using children's instruments can also be insulting to adult sensibilities, unless the adult and a child are using them together as intergenerational play. Music stores sell shakers without handles that are small and egg-shaped, and can easily be held in the palm of the hand. These egg shakers are quite popular and produce a good sound.

The tambourine evolved from the drum, to which jingles were added around the perimeter. I prefer to use a tambourine that has a skin over the center rather than the type without a skin for a couple of reasons. First, the skin offers more surface area to be tapped or touched, and second, the instrument can either be played like a drum or shaken. Tambourines without skins can be shaken or tapped against something, but cannot be hit with a mallet or drum beater owing to the lack of surface area. Try out different types and see which kind you prefer. Again, take into consideration size and sound quality. Some skins are made of high-quality human-made fibers that can be cleaned easily. Other skins are natural fibers that may change pitch or dry out. Still others are made of a poor-quality plastic that sounds tinny.

Claves (pronounced *klah-vays*) are similar to rhythm sticks, only wider and slightly louder. They are of Latin origin, and generally made from wood. Claves require the use of two hands, and are played by hitting them together. If the resident is unable to use both hands or has some difficulty getting the motion, claves can be shared between two people.

Hand drums are useful and appealing to many. They come in many sizes, although typically about the size of a pie tin. Hand drums may also be played with a beater or a mallet of some kind. Before using hand drums, examine the condition of the resident's hand. Sometimes the older person's skin is fragile, and striking an object with the hand may cause pain. Arthritis also can inhibit a person's ability to use the drum and other instruments. Watch for facial expression, especially if the resident is unable to tell you when she or he is experiencing pain. If it's not possible for the resident to use her or his hands to strike the drum, be prepared with a drum beater or mallet. Try out different drum beaters, since they come in a variety of sizes and densities. A hard plastic mallet is going to be much louder that a felt- or yarn-covered mallet or drum beater.

You're probably familiar with these percussion all-stars: the bongos. Bongos are two small drums, connected by hard plastic, metal or wood. One drum is larger than the other, so that bongos produce two different pitches. A more recent addition to the drum world are paddle drums. They are named for their shape, which looks like a paddle, and are lightweight with a sturdy handle. They are available in a variety of sizes and come with a mallet. An ocean drum is a completely enclosed drum filled with small beads that can be shaken or swirled to create a sound reminiscent of the ocean. Ocean drums are often visually appealing, with one side colorfully decorated, and the other made of clear plastic so that the beads can be seen.

Drums are excellent for sharing. They can be played simultaneously or alternately. Here is a list of suggestions. Add your own ideas to this list!

FIFTEEN WAYS TO MAKE A RHYTHMIC CONNECTION

1. Try having a conversation without using words by tapping on the drum.

2. See if the resident can copy a simple beat or pattern.

3. Try beating out the rhythm of your names, and then repeat it to make a pattern.

4. Try suggestion 3 with favorite foods, short phrases, names, any topic of interest.

5. Scratch the surface of a drum lightly with your fingernails.

6. Imitate the sound of a heartbeat.

7. Tap fingers lightly to sound like raindrops.

8. Start softly and slowly, gradually building to a fast crescendo.

9. Play loudly and gradually fade out.

10. Combine suggestions 8 and 9.

11. Play the "boom boom clap" of "We Will Rock You" by Queen.

12. Try to hear different pitches in different parts of a drum.

13. Turn over a hand drum and use it to carry your other small percussion instruments.

14. Turn a rain-stick over gently and listen to the rainfall.

15. Play rhythms you hear in the environment: the *chugga-chugga* motion of a train; the agitation of a washing machine; the ticking of a clock; the wind beating a flag or causing something to click steadily.

Other percussion instruments of interest include the triangle, jingle bells, woodblock, rain-stick, chimes, gongs, and cymbals, to name a few. Depending on the interest and culture of the person in need of care, you can make your selections accordingly. You may be able to borrow a variety of instruments to determine which seem appropriate for your particular situation, then only purchase the instruments you and your resident are really attracted to. If you are working with residents in a community-living arrangement, a small collection may be shared among all the residents.

YOUR PERSONAL TOUCH

There are two more elements of music that play an important role in how it sounds, and that give it the personal touch and flexibility that you can enjoy when playing "live" or singing along with recorded music. The first element is the tone-color or "characteristic sound" (Crowe 2004, p.69) of the specific instrument or voice creating the music. The other is the dynamic shading of music—the volume and rate of speed at which you play. These elements offer great variation, and are responsible for much of the musicality in playing and singing of music. You may think of it as your chance to be the conductor—you decide how fast to go, how loud or soft to sing, and when to change direction!

The tone-color of music may be velvety, like "the fog-horn" voice of Mel Torme, or harsh, like a cymbal. Each instrumental and human voice is distinct and unique, and like our speaking voices, each singing voice is different. It is your personal sound that is so important in connecting with others, and that is most likely to provide comfort to someone with dementia. Dynamics are loud or soft, sustained or short, but so much more in between. They are what make music come to life—the hush of a lullaby, the romantic ebb and flow of a love song, the crispness in a march. This is where natural musicianship and feeling make up for technical ability. Think of people who don't have a classically beautiful voice, or even a trained voice, but are deeply treasured for their unique sound and sense of style: Ethyl Merman, Louis Armstrong, and Bob Dylan are just a few.

Anyone with a sensitive ear can incorporate the fluctuations in music that make it more varied, flexible, and interesting, even if it's the same song being repeated frequently. By alternating tone-color—quietly one time, lively the next—and rate of speed, familiar music remains fresh and appealing, just a little different every time. Because of these simple variations that you can include in your music-making from the very beginning, your own singing and rhythm is going to be appreciated for its personal appeal and ability to be changed in the moment.

MOVEMENT TO MUSIC

I found in my work with people who have cognitive processing issues that using something physical at the beginning helped to bring them into the moment and helped them to realize that something new or different was happening. It really depends on the person and severity of the illness. Sometimes physical touch is the best way to help someone recognize that you are there, and gentle movement can be the most engaging activity to do with music.

The following is list of ideas to begin moving to music. All of these are intended for seated movement, and they are meant to be repeated only a few times. Always make sure that your resident is physically able to participate in simple seated movement by asking his or her healthcare provider. Any time a person raises arms above chest area, there is more work placed on the heart, so only repeat motions over the head a few times. It is best to do a motion once or twice, then listen to the music or sing along, then repeat a movement, instead of doing continual movement. The purpose of the movement is to raise awareness of self and the environment, not to do physical exercise. It is generally most effective if you model the movements for the resident, facing him or her, and sitting down at eye level. Modify movements to match the ability of your resident.

TEN WAYS TO CONNECT THROUGH MOVEMENT

1. Yawn and stretch like you do when you wake up. Try some classical favorites, like Vivaldi's "Four Seasons" or use nature or environmental sounds. Breathe deeply and stretch again, picturing your favorite scene in nature. You may enjoy looking at a picture of a nature scene, talking about what is in the picture, then yawning and stretching again.

2. Alternate arms, reaching upward as if climbing a ladder. Try the music, "Jacob's Ladder" or "Climb Every Mountain." Add in leg motions for climbing if you desire.

3. Continue moving legs as if walking or marching. Try, "Walk of Life," by Dire Straits, the Johnny Cash song, "I Walk the Line," or Nancy Sinatra's, "These Boots Were Made for Walking" to get in the rhythm.

4. Remaining seated, move your body from side to side, reaching your arms out to the sides. Next, reach forward and back, which may be done with a partner, holding hands facing each other and pulling the other person gently toward you, then switching direction. For fun, sing "Row Your Boat" as you rock back and forth.

5. Try swimming to music. Do the motions of the crawl, the breaststroke, the backstroke, whatever you like. Then, hoist the sail, row the boat, do any

nautical movements you can think of. Fun music can include old sea shanties, like "Blow the Man Down" or something more modern like a tune from the Beach Boys. Ahoy, mate!

6. Do the "Twist" and all the fun moves of the 1950s. Try the "mashed potato," the "shoulder shrug," the "monkey," the "hand jive," anything goes! Move to the music of the movie "Grease," or you can use recordings of your favorite 50s artists, like Elvis Presley or Jerry Lee Lewis.

7. Get back to nature by moving in the gentle arc of a rainbow, drifting arms like clouds, and moving fingers like rain falling. Nice music for this is, "Hawaiian Rainbows" or "Over the Rainbow." Use a rain-stick for added effect.

8. Making hand and arm movements that embody the song text is a wonderful way to move expressively to music, and may be abbreviated or modified to your needs. Start with a song that has a few words with lots of repetition, and make up just a few motions to depict the words. You may decide to use some signs taken from sign language, and these can be very helpful in communicating with the deaf or hard of hearing. See the Resources section in the Appendix for websites on sign language.

9. Move like a belly dancer to Middle Eastern music! This can be fun with a scarf or finger cymbals (zils) for added drama.

10. Do the steps of ballroom dancing with your feet. Try the 1–2–3, 1–2–3, of a waltz ("Blue Danube," "Skater's Waltz"), the tango ("La Rosita," recorded

by Laurindo Almeida/Charlie Byrd), the cha-cha ("Smooth" and "Oye Como Va," both recorded by Santana), whatever you like! Be sure to play music that matches the dance. There's always the "Macarena!"

HARMONY

Harmony is often considered the support of the melody, and usually is the part played on the piano, guitar, or other accompaniment instrument. It is what happens when more than one note is played or sung at the same time, and adds to the emotional element of a piece of music (Crowe 2004). Many churches use harmony as part of the worship music, from choirs to organs to gospel music, and we have become accustomed to hearing harmony as an accompaniment and addition to melody. Since many people are able to play a harmonic instrument and may have one in their possession, I have included the chords for popular songs at the end of this book. These chords are the basic harmony that can accompany singing. The keys that are used on the song sheets provided in this book should be in a fairly comfortable singing range for most adults. There is also a variety of resources available for self-teaching in music in the form of videos and DVDs, songbooks and CDs, and accompaniment in the form of karaoke or "Music Minus One" which may be purchased online or in a music store. See the Resources section in the Appendix for some suggestions.

2

SINGING AND CHOOSING SONGS

BECOMING COMFORTABLE WITH YOUR VOICE

Most people are born with a natural ability to speak and sing. Singing is a joyful expression of the human spirit. Some people are more comfortable with using their voice than others, but the vast majority of us are able to carry a tune. One of the first considerations is finding where our natural voice lies. For females, the higher singers are soprano, the lower voices are alto. Men's voices are tenor and bass, with bass being the lower of the two. The main thing is to sing in the register of your voice that is most comfortable. Depending on your mood or the time of day, your voice may change. Don't be alarmed—it is normal for your voice to be a little lower in the earlier part of the day.

Summarizing the music therapy research on various aspects of singing among people who have severe cognitive impairment, Clair (1996) indicates that singing in a lower key that has been slowed down makes it much easier for the person with dementia to be able to participate. Live music is preferable to recorded so that adjustments may be made to pitch and tempo, and the voice of a familiar person is usually the preferred voice for the person who has dementia.

Singing may be thought of as an extension of speaking. The only difference between singing and speaking is that when you sing, you must hold out a tone longer, and fluctuate your voice between higher and lower pitches. The pitch is how high or low the note is that is being played or sung. A high-pitched instrument is a piccolo, a low-pitched one is the tuba. On the piano, the lowest pitches are to the far left, and the highest on the far right. We fluctuate our voices between pitches when we are speaking, although not to the degree that pitches change when we sing. When someone doesn't fluctuate vocal pitch much, it is called "monotone" which is not very common. Usually the more excited someone is, the higher the pitch of his voice. Someone who is sleepy or depressed will have less inflection, and may have a lower-pitched voice than when that person is wide awake or cheerful. Different languages and cultures require different uses of pitch. For example, Chinese languages use the same combination of vowel and consonant but change pitches to change the word meaning. In some other languages, there is very little inflection or fluctuation in pitch at all.

We use the same apparatus when we sing as when we speak: breathing and letting out sounds, then using our lips, teeth, and tongue to form words. For some confused people, just making sounds may be easier than conversing, particularly in the middle and even sometimes in the later stages of dementia (Peters 2000). Making sounds is a valid form of expression, and we can learn something from the type of sound a person makes. It is helpful for you to become comfortable with making sounds, even if the sounds are not musical or pretty. The way to become comfortable is by experimentation and repetition. By vocalizing frequently, it will begin to feel natural.

There are a few reasons to learn and practice warm-ups leading to singing. The first is to get comfortable with making sounds other than singing. Some people with cognitive deficits will make sounds that are not words or easily understood tunes, but may be bits or fragments of words or songs. If you have learned to become comfortable making a variety of sounds, you will have more opportunities for interacting. Another reason for exercising the voice is to increase your comfort level as a caregiver. When working with sound, it is inevitable that others will hear you. If you have done vocal play many times, you will be more comfortable, confident, and relaxed when singing or making sounds with your resident, and less likely to feel self-conscious when overheard. When you are comfortable and confident, the person with whom you are interacting will feel more secure, enabling greater trust between you. Repetition of vocal exercises will make vocal production so commonplace that you won't have to focus your attention on your singing; you can focus on the resident's reactions and responses to the music you make together. Naturally, warming up your voice helps it to be more flexible and limber for singing. Just as we stretch out our muscles as preparation for exercising, it is helpful to prepare the voice and breath for singing.

Singing and practicing of vocal warm-ups is also very valuable to the care provider. The act of singing involves deeper breathing and concentration than everyday speech.

It is not just the person with dementia who may be under stress, but you as well (Bonner 2005). Since the benefits of singing are an increase in deeper and more "conscious" breathing, relaxation and physical stimulation are benefits that can be received by you as well as the recipient of your care (Clair 1996).

The following vocal exercises may be used to help warm up your voice and develop breath control. I have learned them over the years from voice teachers and choral directors, and through experiences working with different vocal sounds with my clients and residents, and with music therapy students. If you want to approach this less formally, or if you don't always have the time to set aside for exercises, just warm up your voice and body whenever you have a few minutes. I often hum along with the radio to warm my vocal cords, and do a few deep breaths, shoulder shrugs and neck rolls as I take mini-breaks through out the day. They are rejuvenating and may be built right into your existing schedule.

DEVELOPING YOUR BREATH CONTROL AND VOICE

The exercises below are for you to warm up with and develop your voice. Try to approach them in a lighthearted and playful way. If they seem like something your resident might enjoy, by all means do them together.

The first three exercises are to help bring greater awareness of breath and develop breath control. Breath control is the ability to take in a large amount of breath and let it out slowly. When singing, a person with greater breath control is able to sing longer phrases without taking a breath. From a therapeutic aspect, deeper breathing helps to develop lung capacity and provides more oxygen to the blood. It also helps to relax the body and mind. Always take a slow, deep breath before singing. It is best to sing from the deepest part of your belly, using the muscle called the diaphragm. The third exercise listed below (Cleveland Clinic Foundation 1995–2008) describes an exercise for diaphragmatic breathing for improving lung health, and is also a wonderful way to improve singing and overall health. The last three exercises listed help to develop your sound production and ability to shift easily between notes.

HISS LIKE A SNAKE

Take a deep breath and let the air out slowly between your teeth making a "sss" sound like a hissing snake. Put one hand on your stomach to feel it expand when you breathe in and contract as you force the air out, and the other hand on your chest, keeping it as still as possible. Breathe deeply and slowly, and repeat two or three times, increasing to five times.

LAUGHTER IS THE BEST MEDICINE

Breathe in deeply and let out your breath on "Ho Ho Ho." Feel your belly bounce as you make the sound. (You can get your inspiration from Santa.) Repeat on "Ha Ha Ha," "Hee Hee Hee," "Hoo Hoo Hoo," and "Hay Hay Hay." As you get more comfortable, increase to four of each, then five of each.

BREATHING FROM THE DIAPHRAGM

Lay down on your back, or sit up straight and relaxed in a chair, and put one hand on your belly, the other hand on your chest. As you breathe in through your nose, feel your lower abdomen push out against your hand while it fills up with air. Try to keep your chest as still as possible against your other hand. Breathe out slowly through pursed lips, pushing your abdomen in as you force out the air. Repeat this for several minutes, and increase the amount of time spent breathing as your diaphragm develops. It helps to close your eyes and imagine your abdomen is a balloon filling and emptying as you breathe in and out.

THE SIREN

Imitate the sound of an ambulance siren, sliding your voice from the lowest pitch you can sing all the way up to the highest pitch, and back down again. Sing lightly, and be careful not to strain your voice. Repeat two or three times, slowly, breathing in deeply before each siren.

ME, ME, ME

Pick a comfortable note, in the middle of your singing range. Any note will do. Hold the "mm" of "me" on this note, feeling the vibration in your nose as much as possible. Open your mouth to let the "ee" sound out, allowing it to be nasal. Alternate between the "mm" and the "ee" in me, opening and closing the lips. Sing three "Mm–ee"s slowly on each breath. Inhale deeply and repeat five times.

HUMMING

Pick a song you know and hum the tune, breathing deeply each time you need breath. Now, take the same tune, and instead of humming, part your lips and sing the tune on "ah" or "oh." Sing the same tune again on "la" or "loo" or your syllable of choice. Finally, sing the song through with words once or twice.

If you notice any pressure or discomfort on your throat while you are warming up or singing, try to adjust what you are doing. Sometimes inducing a good exaggerated yawn helps to relax everything. Vocalizing and singing should never hurt! Only sing in ways that are comfortable and pain-free. The main cause for pain is tension, so the more relaxed you can become prior to singing, the easier it is going to be. Some people find it helpful to check the mirror to see if any muscles, like the jaw or lips, are being held tightly, or to see if the head is being held in an awkward way.

CHOOSING SONGS AND SINGING THEM

Choosing songs can be simple. Begin with the most popular and common songs you can think of. "You Are My Sunshine" is a song almost everyone knows. "Happy Birthday" is a perennial favorite, and you can always think of someone's birthday to sing about. You can use a birthday of a famous person or celebrity as a way to work in an interesting fun fact, even if you are the only one who can appreciate this. It is important to keep your own morale up, and any fun tricks that add a smile to your day are worth the effort. Include songs that the person you are caring for has enjoyed, particularly from his or her young adult years. Introduce the songs one at a time, and see what songs seem to garner the best reaction.

There are many songbooks and recordings compiled according to decade, and many artists have become associated with a specific era or style. Movies, Broadway musicals, and dance crazes are often a good place to begin the search for music that will be familiar. Be aware of cultural and religious affiliations because many people have strong ties to heritage. Even if a person has never been extremely musical, she will probably remember the popular music from her youth, or worship music, or a courtship or wedding song. By offering choices, you help to make a connection with the resident's past, and help to fill in some of the gaps that the memory may have left out. There is a song list in the Appendix (Jackert *et al.* 2003) that you may find helpful.

If you are unfamiliar with your resident's own collection of music, use recordings and sing along with them until you have learned them. You can always use recordings for background, but *most often it is the use of your own live voice that elicits the best response.* So, sing along with a recording as best you can until you no longer need it. If the person you are caring for sees you singing along, that person will be more inclined to try. Above all, do not worry if you don't sound like the singer on the recording. A "professional" sounding singer could be intimidating, and may actually inhibit the person you are caring for. Do pay attention to see if you are singing in the same key as the recording. This will help you to develop your ability and recognize when the pitches you are making are accurate. Sometimes, especially when a female is trying to sing along with a male, and vice versa, it is nearly impossible to match your voices. Try to find a recording of someone of your own gender and vocal range to sing along with. Experiment with different styles for fun and flexibility.

It also helps to sing music that you, the caregiver, are familiar with. This will give you extra confidence and feeling in your singing. Pick music that you enjoy, and do your best to find songs that are appealing to both yourself and the person you are caring for.

While you are singing with the resident, encourage him to sing along. If he is able to read, have a large-print song sheet available. Only supply one song sheet at a time to avoid confusion. Notice if the song seems too high or too low for the voice range of the participant, and adjust it if you are able. Try to imitate the sounds of the resident. If he is humming, hum with him instead of using the words. You can try adding words later, but don't be afraid of singing "la" or "oo" if that is all the person is able to do.

There is also benefit in singing *for* someone else. Even if someone is unable to respond, unless there is profound hearing loss, he is still hearing your voice. Even with a hearing loss, leaning in close to someone and singing to him will generate warm feelings and enhance the mood and environment. There are vibrations produced when we sing which can be felt in the body of both the singer and the listener. The only time it's important to *not* sing is if the music-making seems to disturb or distress the person you are caring for in any way.

THE IMPORTANCE OF REPETITION

Repeat each song for as long as it seems interesting to the resident. You can change the tempo (rate of speed), make up words appropriate for the moment, sing while keeping the beat with percussion, and experiment in ways that are comfortable to you. If you get a positive response from a particular song, use it each time you meet. A music therapy pioneer, Edith Boxill (1985) calls this the "Contact Song," which means exactly what it says. It is a certain, special song that captivates and brings you, the caregiver, in contact with the person you are bringing music to: music that makes a positive connection. It is typically the song where musical "contact" is first gained, when other music does not seem particularly meaningful. The significance may be as simple as that it is a song that is recognizable and familiar, particularly when memory is fading and so many things seem unfamiliar. Its meaning may be in an association with a particular person or event. In the case of my grandmother, it was the music of her native language and country of origin. There have been times when the most important song was the one with the person's own name in it, like "Mary" or "Peg of My Heart" or "Bill." Sometimes the meaning or significance is not clear, but the obvious enjoyment and pleasure *are* clear, so we repeat the song.

When the person you are caring for sings or makes any attempt at vocalizing, make sure to provide positive feedback, with words, gestures, and repetition of the music that is eliciting this response. You can show your pleasure at the resident's involvement by smiling, clapping, and praising her efforts. Introduce different songs throughout the sessions, always making a mental note of those the resident enjoys. Include favorites of your own from time to time. Your enthusiasm can be contagious. Keep track of "core songs" to be used at each music visit, and vary others according to season and mood.

Many people like to use the same opening and closing music each session to maintain a structure. Chances are this will be a reassuring format for you to try, and will help both you and your resident with the transition of beginning the visit and ending it. Since the spoken word is not necessarily understood, these simple patterns and rituals can help with ordering the world of the person with dementia as well as the person caring for her.

There are ways to alter familiar music to keep it fresh and interesting, like adding percussion, using movement, singing with and then without a recording, and altering tempo and dynamics. In an article "Repertoire recommendations by music therapists for geriatric clients during singing activities" (Van Weelden and Cevasco 2007) popular music received the greatest number of song recommendations, followed by songs from musicals, hymns, and, finally, patriotic songs. Most people prefer the music from their young adult years, and this is most ingrained in their long-term memory. If you can find the specific music liked by the particular individual you are caring for, that is best. If you are not sure what the person you are caring for liked, use popular music from their time as a young adult, between 18 and 30 years old.

3

MAKING A
CONNECTION

The first few music visits you have with your resident or loved one will be a time of getting to know each other musically, and will offer you the chance to make an informal but important assessment. As a caregiver, you need to determine the abilities and interests of the person in need of care. You will likely already have some knowledge of this person, either as a staff member who has had occasion to work with this resident, or as a relative or friend. If it is helpful, copy the following pages as needed and write directly on them. They can be your own data recording sheets to track your progress.

HOW TO START

BEGIN THE SESSION BY SAYING "HELLO" AND CALLING THE RESIDENT BY NAME

It is usually most effective to use the resident's first name, since this is most deeply ingrained in the memory. However, if you are a family member, you will probably be most comfortable with the title you have been using for many years—"Grandpa," "Auntie," and so on.

If you are younger or from a more formal culture, you may prefer to call your resident or loved one by a title (Mr, Mrs, Dr, and so forth) or you may have specific guidelines if you are working for a facility.

INTRODUCE YOURSELF AND STATE YOUR PURPOSE

"My name is Robin. I am here to play music with you." It can be very difficult for a family member whose relative no longer recognizes them. If this is the case, tell the person gently who you are, and what your relationship is. "Hi, Grandma, this is your granddaughter Robin. I came to visit and sing songs with you."

If you do not notice any response, call the resident's name again, gently moving his hand or shoulder. *Never come up behind someone and put your hand on him, as moves from behind may be frightening or disorienting.* Make as much eye contact as the person allows.

NOTICE RESPONSES OR REACTIONS
Verbal content and clarity
If a response is verbal, is it appropriate? Are the words clear and meaningful? Unclear? Are you hearing only fragments of words, or words in an earlier language?

. . . .

. . . .

. . . .

Vocalizations
Are any sounds being made that aren't words? Do the sounds seem to have communicative value? If so, can you tell what meaning is being conveyed? Can you hear tension? Anger? Calm?

. . . .

. . . .

. . . .

Eye contact
Is the person you are caring for looking at you or moving his head toward the direction of your voice? Does eye contact come and go? Are eyes closed? Are they open, but not focused?

. . . .

. . . .

. . . .

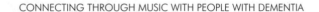

Facial expression

Are facial expressions showing tension? Happiness? Sadness? Anger? Agitation? Confusion? Are expressions changing or remaining the same? Notice also the level and intensity of expression, for example no noticeable expression at all.

. . . .

. . . .

. . . .

Body posture

How is the person you are caring for positioned? Does he look comfortable? Is their body relaxed or tense? Does he seem to be in control of their body? How do his hands feel when you shake them? Warm, dry, cold, clammy? Can you tell if he is able to use both hands, or if he favors one hand?

. . . .

. . . .

. . . .

Movement

Is the resident's body moving or still? Are there any tremors or shaking? Is she walking or seated? What are the possibilities for physical movement? Foot tapping, hand and arm movement or head-nodding, should all be noticed.

. . . .

. . . .

. . . .

OPENING SONG
BEGIN WITH A SONG YOU THINK THE RESIDENT MIGHT LIKE
Take the hands of the resident and sway gently to the music. If the resident is able, invite her to dance, and assist her in moving around the room. A seated dance is often the best choice, if a person's stability is in question. Use a recording if you like. Use music from the resident's country of origin and from her teenage and young adult years.

AS THE MUSIC PLAYS, NOTICE THE RESPONSE

- Verbal or vocal.

- Eye contact and expression.

- Movement.

Is there any sign of recognition or awareness? Do you notice humming or speech? Any body movement or change in expression? Is there a change in breathing? Make a note of any responses, or a lack of response.

....

....

....

INSTRUMENT PLAYING
OFFER A MARACA AND DEMONSTRATE HOW TO SHAKE IT
Notice the response, for example:

- Shakes maraca independently.

- Shakes maraca with assistance.

- Resists or pulls away.

- Limp or rigid hand.

Does the resident need total assistance to play the maraca, requiring the caregiver to physically manipulate her hand? Is the resident more comfortable using the right or the left hand? Is there agitation? Does the resident have a physical impairment that inhibits the use of hands? Is there any expression of pain on the face, or a sharp pulling back of the hand that may indicate discomfort? Are the hands swollen or arthritic? Is the resident able to stop and start with a cue from the caregiver? Can she imitate the way the caregiver plays, for example speeding up or slowing down?

. . . .

. . . .

. . . .

TURN ON HIGHLY RHYTHMIC RECORDED MUSIC

Use dance, march, calypso, Latin, reggae or similar. Help the resident play to the beat. Notice the response, for example:

- Plays with rhythm independently.

- Needs assistance to play on the beat.

- Cannot play owing to physical limitation.

- Accepts total assistance from caregiver.

- Resists or pulls back.

Notice if the response is different when music is played in the background, as opposed to when there was silence. Give simple verbal direction, and demonstrate instrument use as frequently as needed. Make a note of any responses or lack of response.

. . . .

. . . .

. . . .

OFFER A TAMBOURINE OR DRUM

Demonstrate how to play it, as you did with the maraca. Try this with just hands first, then with a beater. Notice the response, for example:

- Plays drum with rhythm independently.

- Needs assistance to play on the beat.

- Cannot play owing to physical limitation.

- Accepts total assistance from caregiver.

- Resists or pulls back.

. . . .

. . . .

. . . .

SINGING

SING A VERY SIMPLE OR POPULAR SONG YOU BELIEVE THE RESIDENT WILL KNOW

Sing it through a minimum of three times, unless there is distress. Sing with the words one time, on a vowel sound another time, for example on "la" or "oo". Offer a large-print song sheet if it seems appropriate. Notice the responses, for example:

- Sings clearly using words.

- Sings vowel sounds.

- Hums.

- Moves lips.

- Moves hands or body.

- Changes facial expression.

- Reads words.

. . . .

. . . .

. . . .

HOW TO FINISH

This informal assessment should take between 15 and 30 minutes. If you have not used 30 minutes, repeat any music you have played, or try something different.

Before presenting the last song, tell the resident you will be leaving shortly. Tell her that you will come back and play music together another time. Thank the resident for participating, regardless of the extent of the participation.

ONGOING EVALUATION

Evaluation is an ongoing process that begins at the first visit. It involves noticing and remembering responses of the person you are caring for as music is played and sung. As you are summing up the situation, be aware of any changes in the reaction of the resident from visit to visit. Ongoing evaluation enables you to select music that is most appropriate, appreciated, and beneficial to the success of the music sessions. You can use the checklist provided on the following page for ongoing evaluation. You will become aware of subtle changes if you continue to remain very observant during the music visits.

After noticing these subtle changes, jot down or make a mental note of when they occur. Is the reaction during a particular song or selection? If it is a positive response, can you repeat what you have done to elicit this response again? Through this type of reflection, you can plan your next visit.

Some residents may show progress in alertness and responsiveness with the increase in special attention. Others may not respond as dramatically or as frequently, but may have moments where a connection is made. Over the course of time, however, it is likely that there will continue to be deterioration in your resident's overall condition because of the ways that disease processes affect the body. Since there are no guarantees on the outcome of this work, remember to praise yourself for the efforts you are making. As much as possible, enjoy. Know that you are contributing to the person with dementia in a way that no one else can, and that you are contributing to his quality of life.

CHECKLIST FOR ONGOING EVALUATION

Notice subtle changes in the following:

- Facial expression.

- Body posture.

- Eye contact.

- Sounds or words.

- Initiation, acceptance, resistance, or refusal of physical contact.

- Reaction to percussion instruments.

- Initiation of, or reactions and responses to, singing.

- Breathing—is it shallow? Deep? Strained?

- Muscle tension or limpness and control of movement.

. . . .

. . . .

. . . .

. . . .

. . . .

. . . .

. . . .

. . . .

. . . .

. . . .

4

PUTTING WHAT YOU KNOW TO USE

You will now begin building on what you have learned. You are aware of the resident's capabilities, and have seen which types of musical interaction, if any, produce a positive response. Subsequent music visits will follow basically the same format as when you were gathering information: take the music activities that produced the most positive responses and repeat them. If the resident seems more receptive to singing, use a variety of songs. If he prefers drumming over all other music activities, devote the majority of the time together to rhythmic play. If he only seems to like moving to swing music, let him do that for as much of the visit as he is able, depending on physical endurance. If you are not noticing any overt response or reaction, continue with music activities, altering them slightly from time to time. Remember that responses may be very small, and may take several sessions to happen, or to be noticed. Also remember that as long as a person can hear or feel vibration, he is receiving, and even if he is unable to respond, the music may help him to feel a little bit better. Try a variety of musical selections, but keep the same basic format.

SUGGESTIONS FOR STARTING YOUR SESSIONS

- Shake hands, reaching out to extend your arms in a greeting: very often, physical contact may help to focus a person with dementia on what you are presenting to her, or energize her if she is lethargic. Say "hello" and explain what you are going to do.

- Begin by offering music based on the resident's interest, or by the interest you perceive. This music may be played on a recording, sung, or made up through drumming a rhythm or playing another percussion instrument.

- Seat yourself as close to the resident as you can while still feeling comfortable. Be aware of what distance helps you to achieve eye contact. You may have to place yourself in the resident's line of vision.

- Move the resident's hands to the music, gently swaying the arms, as long as you are fairly confident that the movement causes no discomfort. You can also lightly tap the leg or arm of the resident in time to the music.

- Include as many of the senses in the music-making as possible. Remember that some might respond more to visual appeal, including your facial expression. The look of an instrument, a large-print copy of song lyrics, or a picture of a familiar recording artist may offer a positive trigger. As mentioned above, tactile sensations can be highly beneficial to residents who need increased sensory input to interact more fully.

- Use more inflection in your spoken words than you typically would. Explain clearly what you are doing and what you are inviting the resident to do with you. A good choice for opening music is the resident's favorite song, music with your resident's name in it, or music that describes an attribute of the person, such as, "Ain't She Sweet."

- If the person you are caring for requires eyeglasses or a hearing aid, make sure that they are being used and are in proper working order.

- Provide water for the resident who is able to drink. It's hard to sing if you're thirsty! A moist lemon swab is an alternative for those who have issues with swallowing.

STRUCTURING YOUR SESSION

The following pages give an outline for opening music, movement, singing, introducing instrument play, and ending with familiar closing music. You can keep a basic structure and modify it as desired, putting the activities in any order that seems appropriate. If you and your resident don't care for singing, leave that out and do more instrument playing and movement. If the resident is unable to move, you will rely more on providing music for the resident to listen to, using physical touch for sensory awareness and comfort. If your basic session structure is working, you can keep the overall format the same for each visit, and rotate the music for variety. Some people like to keep the opening and closing music the same each visit to add more structure and familiarity.

SESSION OUTLINE (adapt and modify)
GREETING WITH OPENING MUSIC
I always prepare the resident first before touching, with eye contact and by giving an exaggerated cue. I extend hands toward the resident, encouraging him to take my hand. You can also place your hand on top of your resident's hand, or slide yours under his if he cannot reach out to you or lift his own hand.

MOVEMENT TO MUSIC
This may be as simple as tapping toes and moving fingers. Some people like to conduct with their hand, a pencil, or a baton. Others are able to dance and enjoy the opportunity to stand and move with a partner, or walk to the beat of a familiar tune.

SINGING
It's good to have a list of familiar songs you know and enjoy to refer to in the moment. You can develop your list as you go. You can also keep a list of recordings to share with the resident, if she is able to choose from it. Making choices can be especially empowering for those who may not have many opportunities to choose. It can also be confusing, so be prepared to help as needed.

INSTRUMENT PLAYING
This is mostly percussion, but if you or your resident are able to play another instrument as well, by all means do so! A few chords on a ukulele or guitar make a wonderful accompaniment to singing.

CLOSING MUSIC AND GOODBYE

This is a time to help make the transition out of music time an enjoyable one. Familiar, comforting music is the best, and a clear indication that you are leaving helps to prepare your resident for the change.

MARY'S MUSIC SESSION

GREETING WITH OPENING MUSIC
"Hi Mary, it's so nice to see you. My name is Robin. I hope you're feeling well. I came to visit and sing a few songs with you. Let's sing 'You Are My Sunshine.' I remember how much you like this song. Can you give me your hands?" As I am talking, I am pulling up a chair so that I am sitting knee to knee with Mary, looking into her eyes.

As I gently take Mary's hands I begin singing. I am not getting much reaction at all, and continue to sing "You Are My Sunshine" several times, switching from words to vowel tones, gently increasing the tempo (rate of speed). I change from hand-holding to arm-swaying, and feel no resistance in her arms. The gentle movement seems to be increasing her alertness. With each variation of the song, I am looking to find ways to help Mary make contact. Next, I encourage her to clap her hands with me, helping her as she needs it. She claps on her own once or twice, and I congratulate her with a broad smile. "How does this feel?" I ask. She cannot tell me, but she looks comfortable and more alert, so I finish "You Are My Sunshine" with a big ending, exaggerating the last words of the song and slowing way down as I finish. I repeat the last phrase of the song again even more exaggerated. And the third time I sing the final phrase, I let go of her hands and hold the final note extra long. "Wow! You look like you are enjoying this! You are looking right at me with your beautiful blue eyes!" I smile broadly again as I see more recognition.

MOVEMENT TO MUSIC

"You have been sitting so still. How about if we try to move a bit more? Let's take a deep breath and lift our hands up together. Here, I'll help you." I take Mary's hands and gently lift them to chest height, then back down to our laps. "How was that, Mary? Was that okay?" I notice that Mary is moving fairly easily, doesn't seem stiff, or in any kind of pain, although she needs me to move her arms for her. "Mary, can you try to move your arms up with me?" I ask, while I lift mine up to give her the visual cue. "I'll put on some music for us to move to." I had learned before meeting her that she likes classical music and had enjoyed going to the ballet, so I put on a CD of "The Nutcracker," figuring that she may know it. As the music plays, I talk over it, suggesting ways to move.

"Mary, let's try to move our hands to the music." I move my fingers up and down, turning my hands over, and Mary watches without moving her own hands. I take Mary's hands and go in little bouncy movements at waist height, back and forth in front of us. "Look, our hands are dancing!" I make small talk about the ballet, "The Nutcracker," and keep moving our hands in time to the music. Next, I ask Mary if she will move her shoulders up and down like she's shrugging, and I demonstrate as she watches, but she doesn't seem able to follow. "How about your feet?" I ask, as I point one foot out and bring it back to resting. "Can you move your feet like a ballet dancer?" I repeat the move with each foot, and I see one of her feet move almost imperceptibly. "Yes! You did it!" I exclaim, bringing attention to Mary's movement by pointing to her feet. "Nice shoes. Do you like mine? How are your feet feeling? Let's keep moving our toes." And I continue to demonstrate simple movement, tapping my feet, marching up and down, changing the direction of my feet, and going back to the original toe movement. Throughout the movement portion, Mary is becoming more alert, and more responsive, moving slightly on her own, and watching me as I move.

SKIP SINGING THIS TIME IN FAVOR OF INSTRU-MENT PLAYING

Instead of moving directly into the singing portion of the session as listed in the outline, I introduce the tambourine to Mary with the recording of "The Nutcracker" still playing.

INSTRUMENT PLAYING

The music is more suggestive of movement and instrument playing than it is of singing, and we can sing later. I pick up the tambourine and tap it in the center to the beat of the music, then hand it to Mary. She doesn't take it, so I place it on her lap and gently tap it so that she can feel the rhythm as she hears it jingle to the beat. I have moved in a progression from simpler (holding hands) to more difficult (playing tambourine). I place Mary's hand on the tambourine and as I tap the rhythm, I encourage her to join me. She looks confused. I take her hand and gently assist her in tapping the tambourine. She is receptive, and begins playing on her own. As she seems more and more confident, I choose a small drum for myself and we play together for a little over a minute. The piece of music is ending, and I feel that this is a good time to make a transition to another instrument and a more interactive way of playing. "Mary, I'm going to turn off the CD player. Will you hold this drum and mallet while I do that?" I pass her the drum and mallet, and take out a second mallet for myself. I beat my own drum in a simple repeating pattern and begin to sing the tune of "Let Me Call You Sweetheart" on the vowel "loo loo" and play steady and consistently. As I play and sing, repeating the song several times, Mary intermittently keeps the rhythm on the drum. She plays for a few phrases, then trails off and stops. I give her a light touch under her hand to remind her to play along, and she smiles and continues. I end "Let Me Call You Sweetheart" after the fourth time through, and say, "Let's sing some more. What would you like?" Mary can't say, so I make a few suggestions.

SINGING

"Are you in the mood for some Irish songs? St Patrick's Day is coming up, and I know a few songs you might enjoy. Should we start with 'When Irish Eyes are Smiling?'" I sing this through two times, once with words and once without, while Mary looks at me, not singing, but still aware. She seems to be getting a little tired. I decide to move to the closing song.

CLOSING MUSIC AND GOODBYE

"Well, it's almost time for me to go. I think we should end with our closing song, 'Mary's a Grand Old Name.' That's a perfect song for you, don't you think? Can you try to sing it with me?" I sing her closing song slowly, and exaggerate each time "Mary" occurs in the song. I end it with a slow, big ending, holding the last note in hopes that she will sing the last word with me. She doesn't sing along, but she looks at me and takes my hand, slightly smiling. I consider this to be a communication, and I thank her for her time.

GRANDMA'S MUSIC VISIT

GREETING WITH OPENING MUSIC

"Good morning, Grandma. It's your granddaughter, Robin. I came to visit you. I thought you might like some music today. I remember you always liked to hear Harry Belafonte sing the 'Banana Boat Song.' I brought in the record and a maraca." I turn on the music and begin to play my maraca, then hand it to my Grandma. "Here, Nonna. Shake it back and forth. That sounds great." Once Nonna shows that she can play independently, I play along with a second maraca. We listen to the song together and Nonna sings along on the repeated line only, "Daylight come and me wan' go home." During the verses, I continue to encourage my grandma, giving verbal cues and physical prompts to help her continue playing for most of the song. I suggest, "Try this" and shake the maraca over my head, and on either side of my body. I offer a second maraca so that Grandma can play two at the same time. I can't sing along very well with Harry Belafonte. His voice is out of my range, and he adds a lot of extra notes. Since I am more comfortable shaking the maraca than I am with singing, I only sing the parts of the song I know well and focus my attention on having fun with Grandma, moving the maracas around in time to the rhythm. Grandma doesn't sing much either, but plays the maracas, mirroring what I am doing.

MOVEMENT TO MUSIC

"Grandma, you seem restless today. Can we try moving with the music? I remember 'When the Saints Go Marching In.' I bet you remember this song, too. Let's move around the room while we listen. Here, let me take your hands. You are really moving now! You're doing great!" I guide her, stepping in time to the music. Grandma seems to tire quickly, although she is still restless and looks agitated and tense. I decide to switch to a slower song, an old Italian waltz, "Vieni Sul Mar" (in English, "Come to the Sea"). This suits her energy level better, and the slower movements are relaxing for both of us. We hold hands and move around the room, with me singing part Italian and part "la la la" where I don't know the Italian words. Nonna sings along a bit, and continues to be more relaxed.

SINGING
Since Grandpa plays mandolin, he joins us now to accompany songs while we sing them. We sing the same songs every time. "Santa Lucia" is my Grandma's favorite and "O Sole Mio" is my Grandpa's favorite. We sing them each a few times, and Grandpa adds in verses that we can't remember. Since these are both slow, we like to pick up the pace for the instrument playing. "Funiculì, Funiculà" is lively and always elicits a request to play along on the drums.

INSTRUMENT PLAYING
We sing and play "Funiculì, Funiculà" with me holding a drum for Nonna to hit with a mallet. We speed up the song a little to make it more exciting, alternating back and forth, taking turns hitting the drum. Since we have the drum out and Nonna's favorite Christmas song is "Little Drummer Boy" we play that, although Nonna just wants to listen. She closes her eyes, and we play a little softer, and she sings on "Rum pa pum pum." I can tell it is time to finish, since she is keeping her eyes closed and breathing restfully.

CLOSING MUSIC AND GOODBYE
"Torna a Surriento" is our closing song. It is a goodbye type of song, because it talks of returning.

It is familiar and comfortable, and we generally sing with lots of feeling. But today Nonna seems to need a nap, so we hum a verse of the closing song quietly as we help her to stretch out on the couch for a rest.

Once you have established initial contact with the person you are caring for, continue with music that you think will keep her engaged in the activity. Keep in mind that sometimes all a person may be capable of doing is observing you. If someone is normally unable to be actively engaged in music-making, but is able to focus attention on you visually during your time together, that is an accomplishment. You are making a richer sensory environment that can be appreciated by the person who benefits from the positive attention.

Choosing music and sound activities to continue the session is individualized according to the resident's interests and mood. Mood can sometimes be assessed by facial expression and level of activity. If someone seems to have a lot of energy, even if she is agitated, try to help her to use that energy in a musical way. If she is able to walk, try moving with her to a particular piece of music you think reflects the activity level she is showing.

MR JONES

GREETING WITH OPENING MUSIC

Mr Jones is well known in the care center where he spends his days while his wife is at work. He appears physically fit and sociable, with bright blue eyes and the ability to greet others by nodding and smiling, saying, "Hello, how are you?" and other short phrases clearly and appropriately. It is only after trying to hold a conversation with him that one realizes he has suffered cognitive losses that make it difficult for him to complete a longer sentence. His inflection and gestures are communicative, but the words become scrambled and his intent is difficult to follow.

We start with a favorite greeting song, "Oh, What a Beautiful Morning" and sing the words together. I play a small bongo drum to keep the waltz beat, and exaggerate the words, singing each phrase slowly and clearly. When I sing slowly, Mr Jones is able to sing along. There is a lot of repetition in this song, which makes it easier for him to sing the words. We sing it a few times, and Mr Jones looks happy, but his attention is drifting and he has stood up several times, even though I have encouraged him to sit down and sing along with me. We are seated near the entry to the building, where Mr Jones likes to watch people entering and leaving.

MOVEMENT TO MUSIC

Since Mr Jones is capable of quite a bit of movement and likes to socialize, I suggest that we walk down the hall while we sing. Mr Jones likes lively music, and we begin walking in time to, "I'm Looking Over a Four-Leaf Clover" without the words, singing on the syllable "doot doot" so as to provide a kind of a steady marching sound to our movement, without adding in the confusion of the words. We walk down the hallway singing and nodding to the other elderly people and those who are working in the facility. It seems like fun for Mr Jones to be walking and greeting people with a head nod, and we continue walking with "Yellow Submarine," a song he knows from when his children were teenagers, and it matches his walking gait quite well. We garner smiles as we pass others, and head back to his favorite chair by the entry.

SINGING

"Mr Jones, I brought the words to a song I think you are familiar with. It's 'Take Me Out to the Ball Game.' Here are your glasses. Can you hold the song sheet?" I begin by singing using the words, underlining the large print with my finger to help Mr Jones follow along. After singing the song through two times, I notice Mr Jones has still not begun singing the words, but is humming softly. He is not looking at the printed lyrics. I stop using the song sheet, and repeat the song without words, humming the tune. I repeat the song still another time, using the syllable, "la" and Mr Jones imitates me, also singing "la" for some of the notes, and going back to the words for the last phrase "at the old ball game!" When we finish singing, I compliment him, "Nice singing, Mr Jones, I bet you had some fun at the ball games, didn't you?" I ask Mr Jones for the picture in his wallet that he has shown me many times before, of himself when he was younger, standing next to his son, wearing a ball cap outside a stadium. I talk about the photo and then talk about how the team is doing. Mr Jones doesn't say anything, but he is looking at me and looking at the photo. After a few minutes, I say, "Let's sing 'Take Me Out to the Ball Game' again. I'll play tambourine to keep the beat." After singing the song another time, I put on a recording of the national anthem using a small CD player, and ask Mr Jones if he'd like to stand up. It gives us both a chance to move again, and is a patriotic gesture particularly familiar to his generation. After the song ends, I help Mr Jones sit down and say, "Now they play 'God Bless America' at the seventh inning stretch. Let's try singing along with that. I found a recording of Kate Smith singing it. She was really great, wasn't she? Would you like to look at her picture while we listen? Maybe we can hum along." As we listen, a few other members of the care center stop and listen.

INSTRUMENT PLAYING

"Mr Jones, it's almost time for me to leave. Let's try playing the drum. You can move your hands up and down on the drum to help keep the beat. Why don't we sing 'Show Me the Way to Go Home,' and you can play along. I'm going to help you get started" and I sit next to him so that we are both facing the same direction. I show Mr Jones how to beat the drum with the mallet and hand it to him. We play a steady beat together while I sing, "Show

Me the Way to Go Home." The song ends and we continue to play the steady beat. I sing the song again and say, "Thanks for playing along with me. I hope you enjoyed the music. I will come back next week and see you again. Let's have our closing song now."

CLOSING MUSIC AND GOODBYE

"Mr Jones, I have to be going soon. Why don't we say goodbye with, 'May the Lord Bless You and Keep You.' Don't worry about the words, we can hum the tune together." Since I haven't learned this particular song that his wife has told me he knows and likes, we use a recording of a choir singing and listen together, humming at times. I extend my hands and Mr Jones grabs them firmly, holding them for the duration of the song and after it is finished. We have a good connection and a positive feeling between us, but I am concerned that he doesn't want me to leave. I continue to help provide closure by reviewing some of what we did together, and try to prepare Mr Jones for what he will be doing next. As I'm talking, I take my hand back. "It was nice to spend some time with you. I enjoyed hearing you play the drum. We'll have to do that again next time. I'll see you next Tuesday before lunch. Would you like to watch TV with your friends?" He says "no." "How about a drink of water?" I get him a cup of water, which has become our routine at the end of the session. It is another cue that our time together is ending. "Janet will be coming to take you into the dining room in half an hour for lunch. Your wife should be here around three o'clock, when she gets finished with work. It was fun singing songs together. Take care Mr Jones, and I'll see you next week. Have a nice afternoon. Goodbye for now."

5

STIMULATING AND RELAXING MUSIC CHOICES

Two very broad categories of music are stimulating music and relaxing or sedating music (Clair 1996). When you are concerned with enhancing or altering someone's mood or activity level, these concepts are of great importance. If a person is agitated or upset, you will try to calm her and help her to feel more secure and relaxed. If she is unresponsive or minimally responsive for long periods of time, your goal is to help her to be more awake, aware and active—in short, to help her participate in her own life. The point is to use common sense when choosing music. Use exciting, stimulating music to help arouse the lethargic person, and play soft, sedating music to calm the overactive and anxious person.

How can you tell which songs will soothe, which will exhilarate? To start, you can be the gauge. Experiment with different recordings and styles of music and notice how they make you feel: your resident will probably have similar reactions, though be prepared to adjust and personalize your choices as you go along. As much as there are norms, there are exceptions. Some people find jazz relaxing, but not everyone. Some people do not like particular sounds, such as a stringed instrument being bowed, or an operatic voice. It does depend on the individual. As part of the disease process, some people may become increasingly sensitive to sound and unable to internally "shut off" background noises like a television or radio in another room, or someone talking on the phone. Minimize all other sounds to help the person with dementia have the most successful music experience possible.

Stimulating music can be found in many styles and varieties. Marches, big band music, dance music from many cultures, rock, pop, and classical all are wonderful examples of stimulating, upbeat music. Sources for sedative music can be found in pop, classical, light jazz, solo instrumental, early music like Gregorian chants, and "new age" music. Your local library can be a valuable resource for recordings and information, and many samples of music may be found online. In a nursing home or senior center, the activities worker or music therapist may have access to a variety of different music. Of course, access to the resident's personal music collection is ideal. Some suggestions are listed in the Appendix.

People who are older and memory-impaired may revert to a first language or music from their youth. It is important not to introduce children's music to an adult, just as we must be careful not to talk to a person in a way that indicates you are talking to a child (Bonner 2005). If, however, the resident initiates the singing of a song from childhood, by all means support the music he is making. When done sensitively and with a cue from the resident, it can be very comforting and reassuring to hear music from childhood. Music from childhood is also very important when young children are present, and can be an excellent way to meet the needs of the elder with memory loss who may still remember and enjoy children's music, while bypassing any "age-appropriate" issue that may surface when only in the company of adults. This intergenerational use of music is a very helpful way to facilitate visits between young grandchildren and grandparents.

When using stimulating or sedating music in a particular situation, it is important to know about the "iso principle" (Crowe 2004), music's ability to match and alter mood. This principle, borrowed and expanded on from psychology, says that when attempting to alter or enhance someone's mood it is generally best to play music that matches the emotional state you believe the person is experiencing, based upon that person's behavior. Then, once you have matched the mood being expressed, gradually shift the person to a more comfortable state by slowly altering the music selections to become either calmer or more vigorous, depending on where you have begun. It makes sense that you would not begin a music session with a loud, rousing marching band piece if someone is half asleep in a quiet room. It would surely frighten and alarm that person, and cause unnecessary stress. In the opposite case, if someone is agitated and aggressive and you proceed with very quiet, gentle music. The person may not hear or notice your input, but if that person does hear it, he or she will probably not feel validated in their distress.

Eloise is pacing in her room, crying and muttering, ringing her hands. I believe her mood is one of frustration and agitation. My first course of action is to do what feels natural, which is to calm her with reassuring words and a calm manner, and playing her favorite song. But as I do this, she has only become louder and more frustrated. According to the iso principle, I play music that is similar to her mood, to gain her attention and let her know that I am aware of her feelings. I choose music that sounds a bit fast-paced with high energy, in her case, the "Battle Hymn of the Republic." I can think of no particular songs that actually sound "agitated" (except perhaps heavy metal or punk, which is rarely appropriate for the older person with dementia) but I am hoping that this familiar song, when sung quickly and with urgency and high energy, may help to capture Eloise's attention.

I play the drum to accompany my singing and mirror Eloise's mood, but I see that the sounds may actually be overstimulating and making the situation worse, so after a minute I put the drum away. I say, "Eloise, let's move together" and sing the familiar refrain of the song, "Glory, Glory Hallelujah" and move my feet to the beat. I want to make it clear that she is safe and in caring hands, and that I want to understand how she feels. I insert the words, "Let's just move around together, let's just move around together, let's just move around together, move around the room." I extend my hands and continue to step up and down in a kind of marching movement. Eloise is beginning to pay attention, so I continue the refrain with my made up words, adding in her name whenever it seems to fit. As Eloise continues to seem more in control of herself, she begins to be a bit calmer, and I gradually slow down the singing and change to "la, la, la" instead of words, then back to the original words.

Over the course of several minutes and several repetitions of the higher-energy song, I gradually slow down and introduce the medium-paced song, "When Irish Eyes Are Smiling." This is a song that I know Eloise is familiar with, and it provides a new mood. I play along with jingle bells, their light sound adding rhythm and changing the mood even more. I then pass the bells to Eloise, and indicate for her to sit down with me. She is now more relaxed and ready to sit, having had some of her energy expelled by the movement, and her attention redirected to something more pleasurable and calming.

The beauty of singing or playing the drum or any other instrument live, as opposed to using a recording, is that you can alter the energy level, speed, and volume to suit the occasion and need. So if you begin a song or beat pattern quickly and loudly, you can bring it down slightly with each verse or repetition of beat pattern. This is true for any song or rhythm that you can produce.

In the opposite scenario, when someone is extremely listless and lethargic, you may begin with very quiet, sedating music and gradually increase the music's intensity, volume, and movement. Treating the resident in a gentle, humane manner indicates you are empathetic to his condition. Physical contact is important to help bring the person into the present moment. Gently rubbing a hand or arm, or patting a knee to the rhythm of a song is a good way to help gain the attention of someone who is sleepy. Call the person by name and ask him to open his eyes if they are closed. Remember that the person may be slow to process what is happening, but with persistence may become more alert and conscious of the environment. Helping the lethargic person to move, both physically and emotionally, slowly and comfortably, to a more desirable mood state and activity level is the goal. Some examples of slower, calmer music are "Danny Boy" and "I've Got Peace Like A River."

There are many medium-tempo songs that may be speeded up, with one of my favorites being, "Hava Nagila." This is an Israeli dance song that accompanies the traditional dance, the Hora, which starts very slowly and gradually picks up pace with the song being repeated several times. It ends with high energy and often, high spirits.

The following are two short vignettes of people who have very low energy and are difficult to engage in music-making.

"Hi Margaret, how are you feeling today?" I ask as I pull up a chair and sit next to her bed. Margaret has not left her bed for over a week. She is not responsive, and is being fed through a tube. "It's Robin. I came to play some music for you." I take Margaret's hand and move it, rubbing her arm. "Margaret, can you open your eyes and look at me? It's a beautiful day. If you open your eyes, you can see the flowers outside your window. It's so sunny and warm." I begin to sing, "Peg of My Heart," and move her arm and hand slightly as I sing. She doesn't seem to notice I am there. I repeat the song, picking up the tempo and singing the tune on "da, da, da," lightly and with a bit more energy. I am hoping the physical contact and sounds will help her to become more alert. I repeat the song another time and go just a bit quicker, and then call her name again. "Margaret, that song was for you, because I know you go by the nickname 'Peg.' Can you open your eyes? I'd like to see your beautiful eyes." I then sing, "Ma, He's Making Eyes at Me" in an effort to help get some more energy, and I strum along on the guitar to give a little extra sound. As I continue to sing the song through the second time, I stop playing and take her hand. She squeezes mine very slightly and seems to move her eyes under her eyelids, but that is the only movement she makes. I decide to sing a more modern song that I know, "Maggie May" by Rod Stewart. I play along on tambourine, and still get no real response, but it cheers me up to sing it, and I imagine that the upbeat sounds may help her to be more aware. I have been visiting for almost 20 minutes now, and I decide to play the closing song, "The More We Get Together" which is a nice traditional tune. I don't know how much my music has reached Margaret, but I am happy to have tried.

The ebb and flow of your visit may be affected by the energy levels of your music choices. Ideally, you want kind of an arc, starting with quieter music, building up energy and engagement as you go, and ending with calm music. Even though making music with someone may not always garner a response, as in the above case, following a simple structure and making a sincere attempt are still valuable. If nothing else, music gives us, the caregivers, an opportunity to spend time with a resident with purpose and intent.

As I enter Douglas's room, he is resting in a large lounge chair. His eyes are closed, and he is breathing heavily. The curtains are drawn and the room is rather dark. I have been asked by the nursing staff to spend some time with him, as he has been depressed since being admitted into the nursing facility. He has fairly severe memory loss, and doesn't remember that he has quite frequent visits from family and friends. I open the shade, turn off the television, and pull up a chair next to Douglas.

"Hello Douglas, would you like to hear some music?" I ask. He mumbles and turns his head away from me. I take his hand and repeat the question, letting him know that the nurses have asked me to come see him. He still does not open his eyes or acknowledge me, so I tell him that I will sing a song for him, if he doesn't mind. I begin singing, "Hello, My Honey," a ragtime song that is normally very lively. Instead of lively, however, I sing it slowly, and gently pat his knee to the beat. He seems to stir just a little, and I sing it again, a bit faster, this time patting his hand. I call his name in between verses, and continue to introduce myself. After I sing the song a third time, I call out his name again with stronger intent, and he opens his eyes. I smile broadly and let him know how happy I am to see him saying "Thank you for letting me come in and share music with you! I have a song called, 'Smiles' that you might like. It's about the types of smiles people have for each other. Would you like to hear it?" I sing the song gently, keeping eye contact, taking his hand again. This movement to the song helps to bring Douglas more into the moment. I sing it a second time more quickly, swaying his arms to the rhythm, and Douglas seems more aware of me, smiling and moving his hand a bit without my help after a while.

Next, I suggest a Polish song, "Melody of Love" knowing that he is of Polish descent, and that the song was popular when he was younger. He brightens considerably when I suggest this, and the chorus is in Polish, which I cannot pronounce very well. I stumble over the words, laugh, and make fun of myself. I show him the song sheet with the large-print words. I sing the song again and ask Douglas to help me with the words. When I reach the refrain, he is able to sing along in Polish, and I repeat it and speed it up a little more, adding energy and volume. I am happy that Douglas has become engaged, and I notice that he has shifted from his lethargic mood to a state of more energy and participation. I continue the music session with recorded music and instrumental play, following the outline suggested earlier (p.67–68).

As you can see, the flexibility in music makes it an ideal resource for helping to shift a mood from underactive to more engaged, and from overstimulated to calmer and more relaxed. These same traits in music also help us, the caregivers, to maintain a calm yet energized mood.

6

MEMORY AND
ASSOCIATIONS

There are many factors that make music a natural choice in helping those with problems related to dementia. The most prominent is the way that music supports and stimulates residual memory. In the book *The Simplicity of Dementia: A Guide for Family and Carers* (Buijssem 2005), a very clear explanation of short-term and long-term memory is given. Short-term memory lasts 20–30 seconds, and is then transferred to long-term memory for our lifetime retrieval needs. When someone has dementia, regardless of the cause, the transfer of information from short-term to long-term memory is disturbed. This transfer of information, the encoding process, cannot take place, and learning new things becomes all but impossible. Things that may improve this absorption of short-term events into the long-term memory are: associations with other known things (I remember my husband's birthday easily because it is the same as my sister's, and both fall on St Patrick's Day); an emotional reaction or enhanced mood (some songs make me feel sad, other's lighthearted, and so on); repetition (music repeats rhythms, harmonies, and lyrics, often simultaneously); organization and categorization of information; the information having meaning (this is unique to the individual listener); and information being provided with humor. This explains a lot of why music can be easier to remember than some other things.

Music itself is patterned and organized sounds, much more organized than typical speech. Remembering a conversation may be hard, but remembering a series of organized notes or a poem is much easier. For example, most of us learned our alphabet to the tune of the "ABC" song, which has the same tune as "Twinkle, Twinkle, Little Star." In addition to the pattern of the musical notes used, with its even phrases and simple, repeated melodic shapes, the song is the already "known" or familiar entity to attach to new knowledge, which, in this case, is the alphabet. To further enhance the memory-aiding features of this song, the letters are organized to rhyme at the end of each phrase. The phrases end with letters "G, P, V, Z" and rhyme with the last word of the song, "me." The song can be repeated many times while a child is learning the alphabet before becoming tedious or boring, and may be sung in a playful and engaging way that brings good feelings with it. It is meaningful to the child, since it is providing pleasure and interaction. So this ABC song matches almost all the suggestions given above that enhance the memory encoding process:

- the song is already familiar or "known"

- the melody, rhythm, and rhyme help to organize the content

- the song can be repeated many times to help solidify the message

- the mood generated is one of playfulness, which will be associated with the learning experience as having a positive mood

- music is engaging by nature, which helps in gaining and maintaining attention.

These elements of music and memory also hold true for older people having the ability to learn and retain information. I have seen people with dementia learn songs that they didn't previously know, and learn how to play instruments that they were previously unfamiliar with. In addition to the memory-retrieval process explained above, it has been postulated that "the brain converts sensory input into waveforms which are stored throughout the central nervous system" (Crowe 2004, p.152). When retrieving a memory, a new waveform that is similar to the one already stored will stimulate the saved memory. This, and the emotional connection and association with music, helps in the retrieval process of memories. In addition to the memories we have stored in our minds, there is also our muscle memory, which is stored throughout our bodies. People who have played a musical instrument can attest to this, describing it as having memory in their hands in addition to their heads. It goes along with the idea that we never forget how to ride a bicycle—the memory is in the body. The same may be said for driving a car, swimming, dancing, or any number of things where the whole body is involved in learning and carrying out an activity.

I have been surprised on more than one occasion when a person who has lost much of her memory seems to remember from week to week how to hold and play a particular instrument, and even learn and repeat a particular melody or rhythmic pattern. The incredible thing about music is that, perhaps because of its holistic nature, requiring many areas of the brain and body to work simultaneously, it can sometimes bypass some of the debilitating condition and allow the healthier parts of the brain and body to take over.

Meg, a member of my resident chorus in the nursing home, had a rich alto voice, and was very accurate in her memory of melodies. She was severely memory-impaired in everything else, and frequently fought with her family, believing that they had not visited her in weeks, when in fact, they visited daily. She also believed she hadn't been given meals because she'd forgotten that she had eaten, so was often distressed and hostile with her caregivers. Meg attended the chorus rehearsals each week, and was able to read the large-print song sheets and play a hand bell when I directed. Setting up for the rehearsal one week, I handed Meg a hand bell with the letter "C" on it for her to play during the song "Oh, What a Beautiful Morning." As I began the song, something didn't sound right. Meg looked up at me and said, "This bell isn't right. I'm supposed to have an 'A'!" Imagine my surprise that she was able to remember that seemingly insignificant detail when so much of her day-to-day memory was no longer accessible. When paired with music, it's simply amazing what some people are able to learn and remember.

Last, and perhaps most importantly, the associations we have with particular songs and pieces of music throughout our lives become deeply ingrained in our memories, especially music that touches our emotions. A first dance, a love song at the time of new love, religious music at an important life event—all these are things that are more fully encoded in our long-term memories, and are easier to retrieve. Peters (2000) cites several authors and researchers who have found that most older adults show a significant preference for music that was popular in their young adult years, when they were between 18 and 30 years old. It makes sense that this time period in life has powerful associations because, for many, this is the time of courtship and marriage, when music plays a vital role in expression of emotion. It is also a time of life when many people go out dancing, and the popular music of the "dance culture" will be closely associated with these good times. If a caregiver is uncertain about what music the resident prefers, it can be particularly helpful to figure out the decade when the person with dementia turned 20, and then find the popular music for that time. Enjoying music from these young adult years may be the most successful way of having a musical memory help someone feel a connection with who she was and she has been.

It is also important to remember that certain music may have an association with a negative experience and not a positive one. There are times when music is paired with something traumatic, such as a significant loss, or an unpleasant event from an earlier time of life.

If such a negative connection with music exists, it is important to educate ourselves as to what music may be upsetting and to avoid it. Although negative reactions may not be common, it is still reasonable to expect a caregiver to do investigation into the history of the person with dementia and learn about the resident's past to ensure that appropriate music choices will be made.

7

CARING FOR YOURSELF

YOUR HEALTH AND HAPPINESS

Caregivers come in all types, personalities, nationalities, and levels of involvement. There are professional caregivers who are helping others for a living. These people have dedicated their lives to working with others, and the job brings many variables to it on any given day. Co-workers may call in sick, a caregiver may have his own family or loved ones to care for, and he may have health issues to deal with as well. There are numbers of residents to care for, other staff to be involved with, families that need emotional support, and personal attachments that develop along the way with those we serve. Having worked in an extended care facility for many years, I have seen the nursing assistants, nurses, social workers, doctors, therapists—all the healthcare staff—take on what seems to be an insurmountable amount of work. All of this while undertaking the very serious and sensitive task of providing care to those with multiple needs.

Now let's look at the caregivers who are not providing care as a career, but are caring for a loved one. It may be a spouse, parent, or loved one who is or isn't related. This brings an entirely different emotional component. There is "history" with this person who suffers from irreversible memory loss, which, like all history, has both positive and negative elements. These caregivers can remember what their loved one was like before the onset of the disease, and have difficulty accepting the changes. There are care-givers who have little respite from caring, and become tired and depressed, wondering why no one else in the family will help. There are adult children who live far away and feel terribly guilty that they can't be more involved in the day-to-day helping of their parent. There are many complex issues related to caregiving, whether it is for a family member or as part of a job.

It is quite natural to need support in the form of counseling, a support group, medical and health-related care, and a social network, whether you are a professional care-giver or a family member caring for a relative. It is also very natural to feel you may not have the time, energy, or "serious enough need" to embark on self-care and self-help projects or experiences while caring for another who is very ill and who has much greater needs. After being in care-giving mode for so long, it is hard to accept help and care for yourself. However, caring for yourself is often the best thing you can do for the person you are caring for. Taking time to evaluate your own personal needs with the assistance of a professional will help to alleviate stress and offer a place to express frustration, grief, loss, anger, and the multitude of other emotions that are a normal reaction to caring for a person who has dementia. Support may come in the form of individual therapy, family therapy, a local support group, an online discussion group, a religious organization, or informal gatherings with others who are in a similar situation. Some caregivers even benefit from music therapy for themselves. There is a listing of music therapy practitioners and health and wellness resources on the American Music Therapy Association website (www. musictherapy.org). Your healthcare provider can give you suggestions on where to find counseling or support groups. The Alzheimer's Foundation (www.alzfdn.org) and the Alzheimer's Association (www.alz.org) can also be a source for support groups, and there are other websites listed in the Resources section in the Appendix. You may find wonderful help and support from a social worker at a facility for people who have memory loss, or a nurse helpline. For music therapists, social workers, psychologists, and some other professionals, supervision is an important aspect of support. This term refers to a mentor, paid professional, or peer who provides guidance for the therapist, helping the student or professional to navigate the clinical world.

Since singing and movement are excellent choices for promoting wellbeing in everyone, I have included some of my favorite physical warm-ups for you, the caregiver. Before singing, I like to do some simple body stretches. The more we are relaxed and aware of our bodies, the more natural and relaxed the singing will be. I encourage you to add in any that you already know and enjoy. If the person you are caring for is able, include him in the warm-ups as well, adapting as needed to fit the situation and people involved. Remember to keep any physical movement within the limits set by your healthcare professional. These movements are meant to be done only a few times in a row, not as rigorous exercise.

BREATH AND MOVEMENT WARM-UPS
ARMS UP
Reach arms straight up over the head, breathing in deeply through the nose, and looking up at the hands as they touch, holding the breath momentarily. Bring arms down to sides, exhaling slowly and loudly through the mouth. Repeat five times.

CHIN DOWNS
Breathe in as you tip your head forward, bringing chin down toward the chest. Breathe out as you roll your head to the left, bringing the left ear down toward the left shoulder. Do not try to bring your shoulder to meet your ear, but relax shoulder down. Breathe in and roll head back to center, chin down towards chest. Breathe out and roll your head to the right, bringing the right ear down toward the right shoulder. Breathe in, roll back to center, and bring chin down toward the chest. Repeat three or four times.

SHRUG IT OFF
Breathe deeply as you pull shoulders up toward the ears. Breathe out, bringing shoulders down and back, with shoulder blades coming gently together. Roll shoulders in circles from front to back several times. Reverse, rolling shoulders toward the front. Repeat this from the beginning two or three times.

FORWARD BENDS
This simple movement helps with awareness of breathing, as well as providing a gentle stretch. Stand tall, feet apart

at hip width, shoulders down and back, knees relaxed and not locked. Breathe in deeply, and on exhalation, gently bend forward, arms dangling loosely. Reach toward the floor, touching toes only if it is comfortable, bending knees slightly as needed. Stay forward for a moment then slowly return to standing, breathing in as you rise. Exhale while standing. Notice your balance. If this is comfortable, repeat twice, focussing awareness on breathing.

HEAD TURNS

Breathe in through the nose and turn your head slowly all the way to the right, focus on an object, and exhale slowly through mouth. Inhale and slowly return your head to center, and exhale. Inhale slowly through the nose and turn your head all the way to the left, focus on an object, and exhale slowly.

YOUR ATTITUDE AND PERSONALITY

Using music with the cognitively impaired older person is both challenging and rewarding. There are times when nothing seems to work. These times may frustrate you and test your patience. On the other hand, there are moments of beauty when a touching connection is made with a person who initially seemed unreachable. People who are willing to do this work, either as a career choice or to help a loved one, are making a statement: "I believe there is untapped potential in this individual. I believe it is possible to improve the quality of life of someone who has severe dementia. I feel that I can help to make the situation better by offering my time, wisdom, talent, and compassion. I can see the human being who lies beneath the illness, and

I want to reach that living soul. I think that a person is capable of feeling, even though he or she may lack the means to express those feelings."

Music can be a new way to help someone express feelings, or just participate more fully in living. As the person offering music, your attitude plays a significant role in affecting positive change. You cannot allow yourself to be easily discouraged. Be confident, not controlling, encouraging but not forcing. Be lively and enthusiastic, remaining calm enough to be able to look for very subtle changes. You must be sensitive to the resident's needs, and be willing to anticipate needs, relying on your own wisdom, intuition, and experience. An impaired person who is confused and cannot speak may still be aware of tension, apprehension, or negativity in another. Do your best to keep a positive attitude. Set the atmosphere and surroundings to be as pleasant and comfortable as possible. An ability to shut out interfering thoughts is helpful, so that you may fully focus on the music session. Your ability to generate a mood of relaxation and fun helps foster a nurturing milieu for the resident, better enabling her to enjoy your time together.

Of course, being genuine is also important. If you are truly sad or frustrated or angry and show it, there is a healing element to that as well, and you should not get in the habit of covering or hiding your emotions. Caring for someone with dementia can be exhausting and emotional work, and it is normal to feel down or be in a bad mood from time to time. It is the *overall* attitude that I am speaking about that should be calm, reassuring, and positive. If you find that more often than not you are frustrated or overwhelmed, take a step back, get help for yourself and your loved one, and re-evaluate your situation with kindness. Be gentle with yourself and use your inner voice as a guide.

USE YOUR RESOURCES!

As a final suggestion, discover and take advantage of your resources. Learn who your supporters are, and go to them as often as you need to. There are many websites, books, and recordings that are available to you. Since time is often a rare commodity, if someone or something is not useful, let it go, and try again elsewhere. There is no perfect match that works for every person. Each person is unique with her own history, preferences, and abilities. Try new things, take risks, and embrace your mistakes, since this truly is where much of the learning occurs. Relish the unknown.

MAKE IT UP AS YOU GO

In music, as in life, there is often no score or script. The term "improvisation" may cause fear and trepidation in the most accomplished actors and musicians, but in reality, each day is a blank slate requiring you to create your moments as they come, one at a time, with you as the author and composer, the improviser. We improvise each time we carry on a conversation, each time we throw together a meal without a recipe, and whenever we forget to bring our music to the session! Dare to be heard even if you are unrehearsed. Forget the suggestion that "practice makes perfect." Practice is valuable, of course. It makes you a better musician and more comfortable with being heard, but you are perfect as you are. Use whatever words suit the song, regardless of whether or not they rhyme. In the moment of being with another, making a musical connection, forget about the past and future, and just be there with the person for whom you are caring.

Dance like there's nobody watching
Love like you'll never get hurt
Sing like there's nobody listening
Live like it's heaven on earth
And speak from the heart to be heard.

William W. Purkey

8

SONGS TO USE

Enjoy this small collection of traditional and popular songs from various cultures. The letters over the song lyrics are chords for those who play a harmonic instrument.

CONTENTS

ALL THROUGH THE NIGHT (AR HYD Y NOS)

Music, traditional Welsh and lyrics by John Ceiriog Hughes (1784).

C Am D G
Sleep my child and peace attend thee,
F G7 C
All through the night

C Am D G
Guardian angels God will send thee,
F G7 C
All through the night

F C F C F
Soft the drowsy hours are creeping

Dm   F G7
Hill and vale in slumber steeping,

C Am D G7
I my loving vigil keeping

F G7 C
All through the night.

C Am D G
While the moon her watch is keeping

F G7 C
All through the night

C Am D G
While the weary world is sleeping

F G7 C
All through the night

F C F C F
O'er they spirit gently stealing

Dm   F   G7
Visions of delight revealing
C   Am   D G
Breathes a pure and holy feeling
F G7   C
All through the night.

AMAZING GRACE

Music, traditional "British Isles" and lyrics by John Newton (1772).

C   F   C
Amazing grace, how sweet the sound
  C   G7
That sav'd a wretch like me!
  C   F   C
I once was lost, but now am found,
     C   G7 C
Was blind, but now I see.
C   F   C
Was grace that taught my heart to fear,
   C   G7
And grace my fears reliev'd;
    C   F   C
How precious did that grace appear,
   C   G7 C
The hour I first believ'd!
C   F   C
When we've been there ten thousand years,

C   G7
Bright shining as the sun,
    C   F   C
We've no less days to sing God's praise
C   G7 C
Than when we first begun.

ARIRANG

Traditional Korean.

D   G D
A-ri-rang, A-ri-rang, A-ra-ri-yo…
D   G   D
A-ri-rang, go-ga-e-ro nu-mu-en-gan-da.
D   G   D
Nareul bu-ri-go ga-esi nue ni-mun
D   G D
Si-bri do mo-gae-sue bal-bung nan-da.

BANANA BOAT SONG

Traditional Jamaican folk song.

Chorus

A   D A   E7   A
Day-O, Day-O, Daylight come and me wan' go home
A   D A   E7   A
Day-O, Day-O, Daylight come and me wan' go home

A

Work all night 'til the morning come

A   E7   A

Daylight come and me wan' go home

A   E7

Daylight come and me wan' go home

Chorus

A   E7

Come, mister tally man, tally me banana

A   E7   A

Daylight come and me wan' go home

A   E7

Come mister tally man, tally me banana

A   E7   A

Daylight come and me wan' go home

Chorus

A

Six-foot, seven-foot, eight-foot bunch

A   E7   A

Daylight come and me wan' go home

A

Six-foot, seven-foot, eight-foot bunch

A   E7   A

Daylight come and me wan' go home

Chorus

A

A beautiful bunch of ripe banana

A   E7   A

Daylight come and me wan' go home.

A

Hide the deadly black tarantula

A   E7   A

Daylight come and me wan' go home.

Chorus

CIELITO LINDO

Music and lyrics by Quirino Mendoza y Cortez (1882).

G   D   G

Ese lunar que tienes

D   G   G/B   D7

Cielito lindo, junto a la boca,

D7

No se lo des a nadie

D7   G

Cielito lindo que a mi me toca

Chorus

G   G7/B   C   Em/B

Ay, Ay, Ay, Ay

D7   G

Canta y no llores

G   G/B   D7

Porque cantando se alegran

D7   G

Cielito lindo, los corazones

HAVA NAGILA

Music, traditional Israeli and lyrics by Abraham Zevi Idelsohn (1918).

B7
Hava nagila
B7
Hava nagila
Em   B7 Am B7
Hava nagila ve nis'mecha
Repeat
B
Hava neranena
        Am
Hava neranena
          B Am   B7
Hava neranena ve nis'mecha
Repeat
Em
Uru, uru achim!
Uru achim be'lev sameach, Uru achim be'lev sameach
Am
Uru achim be'lev sameach, Uru achim be'lev sameach
    B7
Uru achim
Am B7
Uru achim
B7   Em
B'lev sameach

JINGLE BELLS

Music and lyrics by James Pierpont (1857).

D
Dashing through the snow
                          G
In a one-horse open sleigh

O'er the hills we go
 A7   D
Laughing all the way

Bells on bob tails ring
                 G
Making spirits bright
              A7
What fun it is to ride and sing
                     D
A sleighing song tonight

Chorus
D
Oh, jingle bells, jingle bells
Jingle all the way
G   D
Oh, what fun it is to ride
        E7   A7
In a one-horse open sleigh

D
Jingle bells, jingle bells, jingle all the way
      G
Oh, what fun it is to ride
   A7   D
In a one-horse open sleigh

D
A day or two ago
       G
I thought I'd take a ride
        A7
And soon Miss Fanny Bright
       D
Was seated by my side
D
The horse was lean and lank,
       G
Misfortune seemed his lot
    A7
We got into a drifting bank
      D
And then we got upsot

LET ME CALL YOU SWEETHEART

Music by Leo Friedman and lyrics by Beth Slater Whitson
(1910).

```
     E
Let me call you sweetheart
           A        (F#)
I'm in love with you
B7                                        E          B7
Let me hear you whisper that you love me, too
E                                    A        (F#)
Keep the lovelight glowing in your eyes so true
A            E
(A    A#dim    E/B)
Let me call you sweetheart
A      B7    E
(C#    A   B7   E)
I'm in love with you
```

MY BONNIE LIES OVER THE OCEAN

Traditional Scottish.

```
   G              C        G
My Bonnie lies over the ocean,
                           D7
My Bonnie lies over the sea,
      G       C        G
My Bonnie lies over the ocean,
  A7              D7        G
So bring back my Bonnie to me
```

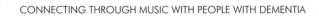

Chorus

G   C A7
Bring back, bring back
    D7   G D7 G
Oh, bring back my Bonnie to me, to me
        C A7
Bring back, bring back,
    D7   G
Oh, bring back my Bonnie to me

G G   C G
Oh Blow ye winds o'er the ocean
             D7
Oh Blow ye winds o'er the sea
G   C   G
Oh Blow ye winds o'er the ocean
 A7   D7 G
And bring back my bonnie to me

Chorus

OH, YOU BEAUTIFUL DOLL

Music by Nat D. Ayer and lyrics by A. Seymour Brown (1911).

 D   B7   E7
Oh, you beautiful doll, you great big beautiful doll.
 A7   D   Em
Let me put my arms about you, I don't want to live

A7
without you.

D   B7   E7
Oh, you beautiful doll, you great big beautiful doll.
          D
If you ever leave me, how my heart would ache.

   B♭
I want to love you, but I fear you'd break.
D   F# Bm D   E   A7   D
Oh! Oh! Oh! Oh! Oh, you beautiful doll!

SANTA LUCIA
Traditional Neapolitan song (1850).

E   B7
Sul mare luccica,
              E
L'astro d'argento
              B7
Placi dae londa,
                E
Prospero e il vento
              B7
Sul mare luccica,
              E
L'astro d'argento
              B7
Placi da e l'onda

E
Prospero e il vento
      A   E
Venite allagile Barchetta mia
    B7   E
Santa Lucia Santa Lucia
    A
Venite allagile
    E
Barchetta mia
   B7   E
Santa Lucia Santa Lucia

SILENT NIGHT

Music by Franz Gruber (1818) and lyrics by Joseph Mohr (1816).

G
Silent night, holy night
D7   G
All is calm, all is bright
C   G
Round yon Virgin, Mother and Child
C   G
Holy Infant, so tender and mild
D7   G
Sleep in heavenly peace
G   D7   G
Sleep in heavenly peace

G
Silent night, holy night!
D7   G
Son of God, love's pure light
C   G
Radiant beams from Thy holy face
C   G
With the dawn of redeeming grace
D7   G
Jesus, Lord, at Thy birth
G   D7   G
Jesus, Lord, at Thy birth

TAKE ME OUT TO THE BALL GAME
Music by Albert Von Tilzer, and lyrics by Jack Norworth (1908).

G   D7
Take me out to the ball game,
G   D7
Take me out with the crowd.
E7   Am
Buy me some peanuts and Cracker Jack.
A7   D7
I don't care if I never get back
        G   D7
Let me root, root, root for the home team,

```
      G              C
If they don't win it's a shame.
               G              E7
For it's 1–2–3 strikes you're out
        A7   D7   G
At the old ball game.
```

TILL WE MEET AGAIN

Music by Richard A. Whiting and lyrics by Raymond B. Egan (1918).

```
     C                    G7
Smile the while…you kiss me sad adieu,
                    C
When the clouds roll by I'll come to you,
F                 C        A7
Then the skies will seem more blue…
D          G         G7
Down in lover's lane…my dearie
C                  G7
Wedding bells will ring so merrily,
               C
Every tear will be a memory,
     F                 C    A7
So wait and pray each night for me,
D      F      G-C
Till we meet again.
```

WALTZING MATILDA

Music by Christina Macpherson and lyrics by A.B. "Banjo" Paterson (1893). Based on a traditional tune.

```
C              G7     Am              F
Once a jolly swagman camped by a billabong,
C         Em       F      G7
Under the shade of a coolibah tree,
        C        G7       Am        Dm
And he sang as he sat and waited by the billabong
C                        G7      C
"You'll come a waltzing Matilda with me!"
```

Chorus
```
C       C7        F      Dm7(Cdim)
Waltzing Matilda, Waltzing Matilda
C            Dm7C   Dm7       G7
"You'll come a waltzing Matilda with me
        C      G7       Am         F
And he sang as he sat and waited by the billabong
C                        G7      C
"You'll come a waltzing Matilda with me!"
```

```
C           G7      Am         F
Down came a jumbuck to drink at the billabong
C           Em         F          G7
Up jumped the swagman and grabbed him with glee
```

       C   G7   Am   F

And he sang as he stowed that jumbuck in his tucker bag

C   G7   C

"You'll come a waltzing Matilda with me!"

WHEN IRISH EYES ARE SMILING

Music by Enerst Ball and lyrics by Chauncey Olcott and George Graff Jr (1912).

G   G7

When Irish eyes are smiling,

        C   G

Sure 'tis like a morn in spring.

C   G

In the lilt of Irish laughter

      A7   D7

You can hear the angels sing

    G   G7

When Irish hearts are happy,

     C   G

All the world seems bright and gay.

       C   G E7

And when Irish eyes are smiling,

        A7   D7   G

Sure they'll steal your heart away.

WHEN THE SAINTS GO MARCHING IN

Music by James Milton Black and lyrics by Katharine Purvis (1896). Based on a traditional tune.

C
Oh, when the Saints go marching in
                                G7
Oh, when the Saints go marching in

          C   C7   F
Oh, Lord, I want to be in that number
          C   G7   C
When the Saints go marching in

C
Oh, when the sun refuse to shine
                              G7
Oh, when the sun refuse to shine
          C   C7   F
Oh, Lord, I want to be in that number
          C   G7   C
When the sun refuse to shine
  C
And on that hal-le-lu-jah day
                      G7
And on that ha-le-lu-jah day

              C7   F
Oh, Lord I want to be in that number
C   G7   C
On that ha-le-lu-jah day

APPENDIX

RECORDING ARTISTS

Here is a list of various artists well-known to older adults. It is a good starting place for finding recordings to use for listening to, singing with, and playing along on rhythm instruments.

The Andrews Sisters
Gene Autry
Count Basie
Harry Belafonte
Tony Bennett
Enrico Caruso
The Chieftans
Natalie Cole
Nat "King" Cole
Perry Como
Harry Connick, Jr
Xavier Cugat
Doris Day
Plácido Domingo
Tommy and Jimmy Dorsey
Deanna Durbin

Nelson Eddy
Ella Fitzgerald
Judy Garland
Billie Holiday
Mario Lanza
Peggy Lee
Glenn Miller
The Mills Brothers
Luciano Pavarotti
Elvis Presley
Louis Prima
Tito Puente
Frank Sinatra
Risë Stevens
The Three Tenors
Hank Williams, Sr.

SOME SONGS USED WITH THE OLDER ADULT

A group of music therapists and I, all with extensive experience playing music with the elderly, compiled a table of frequently requested songs for an educational institute for the American Association of Music Therapy (Jackert *et al.*, 2003, p.27). The composer column lists musical composer and lyricist, when this information is known. Because the group that organized the original list is from the USA, the song list comprises more American music than other nationalities. I have tried to fill in some of the gaps with traditional music from other countries, but there are many more songs for you to find and include that reflect your nationality and interests. We hope you enjoy using these songs as a starting place, and will find even more that are particularly meaningful to the person you a caring for. Tip: Look for songs that were popular in the decade when the resident was a teenager and young adult.

Table: Songs for older adults

Title	Year	Composer (performer)
A Bushel and a Peck	1950	Frank Loesser
After the Ball	1892	Charles K. Harris
Ain't She Sweet	1921	Yellen/Ager
Ain't We Got Fun	1921	Khan/Egan/Whiting
Alice Blue Gown	1919	McCarthy/Tierney
All I Do Is Dream of You	1934	Freed/Brown
All of Me	1931	Gerald Marks and Seymour Simons
All Through the Night	1784	Traditional Welsh

Title	Year	Composer (performer)
Aloha Oe	1893	Queen Liliuokalani
Always	1925	Irving Berlin
Amazing Grace	1800 (lyrics)	Traditional British Isles/ John Newton
America	1831 (lyrics)	Thesaurus Musicus Tune –British/ Samuel F. Smith
America the Beautiful	1895	S. A. Ward/Katharine Lee Bates
April Showers	1921	Sylva/Silvers
As Time Goes By	1931	Herman Hupfeld
Baby Face	1926	Davis/Akst
Back in the Saddle	1938	Gene Autry/Ray Whitley
Band Played On (The)	1895	Palmer/Ward
Battle Hymn of the Republic	1890	William Steffe/Julia Ward Howe
Beautiful Dreamer	1865	Stephen Foster
Beautiful Ohio	1918	MacDonald/Earl
Beer Barrel Polka	1939	Brown/Timm/Seman/ Vejvoda
Blue Hawaii	1929	Baer/Caesar/Schuster
Blue Moon	1934	Rodgers/Hart
Bicycle Built for Two (Daisy, Daisy)	1892	Henry Dacre
Bill Bailey Won't You Please Come Home	1902	Hughie Cannon
Blue Skies	1926	Irving Berlin
Bye Bye Blackbird	1926	Dixon/Henderson

Title	Year	Composer (performer)
By the Light of the Silvery Moon	1909	Madden/Edwards
Caissons Go Rolling Along (The)	1908	Edmund L. Gruber, William Bryden and Robert Danford
California Here I Come	1924	Jolson/DeSylva/Meyer
Carolina in the Morning	1922	Gus Khan
Carolina Moon	1928	Benny Davis and Joe Burke
Chattanooga Choo-Choo	1941	Gordon/Warren
Cielito Lindo	1882	Qirono Mendoza y Cortez
Don't Fence Me In	1944	Cole Porter
Don't Sit Under the Apple Tree	1942	Stept/Brown/Tobias
Down By the Old Mill Stream	1910	Tell Taylor
Dream a Little Dream of Me	1930	Kahn/Schwandt/Andree
Easter Parade	1947	Irving Berlin
East Side, West Side (The Sidewalks of New York)	1894	Lawlor/Blake
Edelweiss	1959	Rodgers & Hammerstein II
Five Foot Two (Has Anybody Seen My Gal?)	1925	Ray Henderson/Sam Lewis and Joe Young
For He's a Jolly Good Fellow	–	Traditional English
For Me and My Gal	1917	Leslie/Goetz/Meyer
Funiculì, Funiculà	1880	Luigig Denza/Peppino Turco
Getting to Know You	1951	Rodgers and Hammerstein II

Title	Year	Composer (performer)
Give My Regards to Broadway	1904	George M. Cohan
God Bless America	1918	Irving Berlin
Good Night Ladies	1847	E.P. Christy
Guantanamera	1966	Jose Marti
Hail, Hail, The Gang's All Here	1917	Estram/Morse/Sullivan
Harrigan	1907	George M. Cohan
Hava Nagila	1918 (lyrics)	Traditional Israeli/Moshe Nathanson/Abraham Idelsohn
Havenu Shalom Aleychem	–	Traditional
Hawaiian Wedding Song	1958	Al Hoffman, Dick Manning, Charles King
Hello Dolly	1964	Jerry Herman
Hey Good Lookin'	1958	Hank Williams, Sr
Home on the Range	1870s	Daniel E. Kelley/Brewster M. Higley
How Much is that Doggie in the Window?	1952	Bob Merrill
I Can't Give You Anything but Love	1928	Jimmy McHugh/Dorothy Fields
Ida! Sweet as Apple Cider	1903	Eddie Munson/Eddie Leonard
I Got Rhythm	1930	Gershwin Bros. (Ethel Merman)
I Left My Heart in San Francisco	1954	George Cory/Douglass Cross
I'll Be Seeing You	1938	Irving Kahal/Sammy Fain

Title	Year	Composer (performer)
I'll Take You Home Again Kathleen	1875	Thomas P. Westendorf
I Love You Truly	1906	Carrie Jacons-Bond
I'm Forever Blowing Bubbles	1918	John Kellette/Kendis, Brockman and Vincent
I'm Gonna Sit Right Down and Write Myself a Letter	1935	Young/Ahlert
I'm in the Mood for Love	1935	McHugh/Fields
I'm Looking Over a Four Leaf Clover	1927	Dixon/Woods
In My Merry Oldsmobile	1905	Bryan/Edwards
In the Good Old Summertime	1902	Shields/Evans
I Saw the Light	1948	Hank Williams, Sr
It Had to be You	1924	Kahn/Jones
It's a Good Day	1950	Harold Arlen, Dave Barbour, Martin Block
It's a Long Way to Tipperary	1912	Judge/Williams
I Think You're Wonderful	1986	Red Grammer
I've Been Workin' on the Railroad	–	Traditional American
I Want to Be Happy	1925	Vincent Youmans/Irving Ceaesar
Jambalaya (On the Bayou)	1952	Hank Williams, Sr
Jeepers Creepers	1930	Mercer/Warren
K–K–K–Katy	1918	Geoffrey O'Hara
Kentucky Waltz	1946	Bill Monroe

Title	Year	Composer (performer)
La Bamba	–	Traditional Mexican
Let a Smile be Your Umbrella	1927	Kahal/Wheeler/Fain
Let Me Call You Sweetheart	1910	Leo Friedman/Beth Slater Whitson
Let's All Sing Like the Birdies Sing	1932	Robert Hargreaves, Stanley Damerell and Tolchard Evans
Look for the Silver Lining	1920	De Sylva/Kern
Lullaby of Broadway	1935	Dublin/Warren
Ma! (He's Making Eyes at Me)	1921	Clare/Conrad
Manana	1947	Lee/Barbour
Marine's Hymn	1919	Jacques Offenbach/Anonymous
May Each Day	1970	Mort Green and George Wyle
Me and My Shadow	1927	Rose/Jolson/Dreyer
Meet Me in St Louis	1904	Kerry Mills and Andrew Sterling
Misty	1954	Errol Garner/Johnny Burke
Moonlight and Roses	1925	Black/Moret
Moonlight Bay	1912	Percy Wenrich/Edward Madden
More We Get Together, The	1912	Madden/Wenrich
Music, Music, Music	1949	Weiss/Baum
My Blue Heaven	1927	Whiting/Donaldson
My Bonnie Lies Over the Ocean	–	Traditional Scottish

Title	Year	Composer (performer)
My Favorite Things	1959	Rodgers and Hammerstein II
My Wild Irish Rose	1899	Chauncey Olcott
New York, New York	1977	John Kander/Fred Ebb
Night and Day	1932	Cole Porter
Oh Susannah	1848	Stephen Foster
Oh, What a Beautiful Morning	1943	Rodgers and Hammerstein II
Oh, You Beautiful Doll	1911	Nat D. Ayer/A. Seymour Brown
Old Folks at Home (Swanee River)	1851	Stephen Foster
On the Sunny Side of the Street	1929	Fields/McHugh
O Sole Mio	1898	Giovanni Capurro/Eduardo di Capurro
Over There	1917	George M. Cohan
Pack up Your Troubles in your Old Kitbag and Smile, Smile, Smile	1915	Asaf/Powell
Pearly Shells (Pupu O Ewa)	1962 (lyrics)	Traditional/Webley Edwards, and Leon Pober
Pennies From Heaven	1936	Burke/Johnston
Polly Wolly Doodle	1880	Traditional
Pretty Baby	1916	Tony Jackson
Put on a Happy Face	1960	Charles Strouse/Lee Adams
Put on Your Old Gray Bonnet	1909	Percy Wenrich/Stanley Murphy

Title	Year	Composer (performer)
Que Sera, Sera	1956	Jay Livingston/Ray Evans (Doris Day)
Red River Valley	1896	North American Traditional
Red Roses for a Blue Lady	1949	Tepper/Bennett
Red Sails in the Sunset	1935	Kennedy/Williams
Roll Out the Barrel	1927/ 1939	Jaromir Vejvoda/Will Glahe
Santa Lucia	1850	Traditional Neapolitan
School Days	1906	Cobb/Edwards
Sentimental Journey	1944	Bud Green, Les Brown and Ben Homer
She'll be Comin' Round the Mountain	1800s	Traditional
Shine On Harvest Moon	1908	Norworth/Bayes-Nor.
Show Me the Way to go Home	1925 (lyrics)	Traditional English/James Campbell and Reginald Connelly
Side By Side	1927	Woods
Singin' in the Rain	1929	Nacio Herb Brown/Arthur Freed (Gene Kelly)
Smile	1954	Parsons/Turner/Chaplin
Somewhere Over the Rainbow	1939	Arlen/Harburg
Springtime in the Rockies	1926	Robert Sauer/Mary Hale Woolsey, Jack Nethersole
Star Spangled Banner, The	1814 (lyrics)	John Stafford Smith/ Francis Scott Key
Sweet Adeline	1903	Harry Armstrong/Richard Gerard

Title	Year	Composer (performer)
Sweet Georgia Brown	1925	Bernie/Pinkard/Casey
Sweet Rosie O'Grady	1896	Maude Nugent
Take Me Out to the Ball Game	1908	Albert Von Tilzer/Jack Norworth
Tennessee Waltz	1947	Redd Stewart and Pee Wee King
Thanks For the Memory	1938	Robin/Rainger
That's Amore	1953	Brooks/Warren
There's a Long, Long Trail A-winding	1913	King/Elliot
This Land is Your Land	1956	Woody Guthrie
Tiny Bubbles	1966	Leon Pober
Tip-Toe Thru the Tulips	1926	Joe Burke/Al Dubin
Too-ra-loo-ra-loo-ral (That's an Irish Lullaby)	1913	James Royce Shannon
Toot Toot Tootsie Goodbye	1922	Kahn/Erdman/Russo/Fiorito
Torna a Surriento	1902	Ernesto De Curtis/Giambattista De Curtis
True Love	1955	Cole Porter
Vaya Con Dios (May God Be With You)	1953	Russell/James/Pepper
Wabash Cannonball, The	1800s	Traditional American
Wait Til the Sun Shines, Nellie	1905	Sterling/Von Tilzer
Walk in the World for Me	1976	Deanna Edwards
When I Grow Too Old to Dream	1934	Hammerstein/Romberg

Title	Year	Composer (performer)
When Irish Eyes are Smiling	1912	Ernest Ball/Chauncey Olcott, and George Graff, Jr
When the Red, Red Robin Comes Bobbin' Along	1926	Harry Woods
When the Saints Go Marching In	1896	James Milton Black/Katherine Purvis
When You Wish Upon A Star	1940	Washington/Harline
When You Wore a Tulip (And I Wore a Big Red Rose)	1914	Mahoney/Wenrich
When You're Smiling	1928	Fisher/Goodwin/Shay
While Strolling Thru the Park One Day	1884	Ed Haley
Yankee Doodle Dandy	1904	George M. Cohan
Yellow Rose of Texas, The	–	Traditional American
Yes Sir, That's My Baby	1925	Kahn/Donaldson
Yes! We Have No Bananas	1923	Silver/Cohn
You are My Sunshine	1940	Jimmy Davis
You'll Never Walk Alone	1945	Rodgers and Hammerstein II
You're a Grand Old Flag	1906	George M. Cohan
You're the Cream in My Coffee	1928	DeSylva/Brown/Henderson
Zip-a-Dee-Doo-Dah	1945	Wrubel/Gilbert

WRITTEN MATERIALS AND SONGBOOKS

The following are some of the best-loved songbooks and music therapy readings for providing music to the older adult.

Birnie, W. A. H. (Ed.) (1969) *Family Songbook.* Pleasantville, NY: Reader's Digest Association, Inc.

Bright, R. (1981) *Practical Planning in Music Therapy for the Aged.* Lynbrook, NY: Musicgraphics.

Bright, R. (1986) *Grieving: A Handbook for Those Who Care.* St Louis, MO: MMB Music.

Bright, R. (1988) *Music Therapy and the Dementias: Improving the Quality of Life.* St Louis, MO: MMB Music.

Bright, R. (1990) *Why Does that Happen?* New South Wales: Music Therapy Enterprises.

Bright, R. (1991) *Music in Geriatric Care: A Second Look.* New South Wales: Music Therapy Enterprises.

Chavin, M. (1991) *The Lost Chord: Reaching the Person with Dementia Through the Power of Music.* Mount Airy, MD: ElderSong Publications.

Hackett, P. (1999) *The Melody Book.* New Jersey: Prentice-Hall, Inc.

Karras, B. (1985) *Down Memory Lane.* Wheaton, MD: Circle Press.

Karras, B. (1988) *With a Smile and a Song.* Mt Airy, MD: Eldersong Publications.

Karras, B. (1990) *Say it With Music.* Mt Airy, MD: Eldersong Publications.

Karras, B. (2001) *Roses in December.* Mt Airy, MD: Eldersong Publications.

Scheldt, K. and McClain, F. (2000) *Guitar Songbook for Music Therapy: A Collection of Spirituals, Children and Folk Songs.* Pacific, MO: Mel Bay Publications.

Shaw, J. (1993) *The Joy of Music in Maturity.* St Louis, MO: MMB Music.

Simon, H. W. (Ed.) (1955) *A Treasury of Christmas Songs and Carols.* Boston, MA: Houghton Mifflin.

Simon, W. L. (Ed.) (1972) *Treasury of Best Loved Songs.* Pleasantville, NY: Reader's Digest Association, Inc.

Simon, W. L. (Ed.) (1984) *Unforgettable Musical Memories.* Pleasantville, NY: Reader's Digest Association, Inc.

Simon, W. L. (Ed.) (1989) *Parade of Popular Hits.* Pleasantville, NY: Reader's Digest Association, Inc.

INTERNET RESOURCES
MUSIC THERAPY WEBSITES

American Music Therapy Association (www.musictherapy.org) or (www.musictherapy.
org/listserv.html for a listing of websites by country).

Association of Professional Music Therapists (www.apmt.org)

Australian Music Therapy Association (www.austmta.org.au)

British Society for Music Therapy (www.bsmt.org)

Canadian Association for Music Therapy (www.musictherapy.ca)

ALZHEIMER'S AND DEMENTIA CARE WEBSITES

Alzheimer's Association (USA) (www.alz.org)

Alzheimer's Australia (www.alzheimers.org.au)

Alzheimer's Disease International (listing of countries) (www.alz.co.uk/help/associa-
tions.html)

Alzheimer's Foundation of America (www.alzfdn.org)

Alzheimer's Society (UK) (www.alzheimers.org.uk)

Alzheimer Society of Canada–Société Alzheimer du Canada (www.alzheimer.ca)

Dementia Care Professionals of America (www.careprofessionals.org)

Ethnic Elders Care Network (USA) (www.ethnicelderscare.net)

Journal of Dementia Care (www.careinfo.org/dementiacare)

SIGN LANGUAGE

American Sign Language (www.nidcd.nih.gov/health/hearing/asl.asp)

ASL browser (http://commtechlab.msu.edu/sites/aslweb/browser.htm)

Australian Sign Language (www.deafsocietynsw.org.au)

British Sign Language (www.britishsignlanguage.com)

European Sign Language (www.europeansignlanguage.net)

REFERENCES

Bittman, B., Stevens, C., Bruhn, K., Westengard, J., and Umbach, P. (2003) 'Recreational music making: A cost-effective group interdisciplinary strategy for reducing burn-out and improving mood states in long term care workers.' *Advances in Mind–Body Medicine, Fall/Winter, 19* (3–4), 4–15.

Bonner, C. (2005) *Reducing Stress-Related Behaviours in People with Dementia.* London and Philadelphia: Jessica Kingsley Publishers.

Boxill, E. H. (1985) *Music Therapy for the Developmentally Disabled.* Austin, TX: Pro-ed.

Buijssem, H. (2005) *The Simplicity of Dementia: A Guide for Family and Carers.* London and Philadelphia: Jessica Kingsley Publishers.

Clair, A. A. (1996) *Therapeutic Uses of Music With Older Adults.* St. Louis, MO: MMB Music.

Cleveland Clinic Foundation (1995–2008). 'Diaphragmatic Breathing.' Available at http://my.clevelandclinic.org/disorders/Chronic_Obstructive_Pulmonary_Disease_copd/hic_Diaphragmatic_Breathing.aspx, accessed August 12, 2008.

Crowe, B. (2004) *Music and Soulmaking: Toward a New Theory of Music Therapy.* Oxford: Scarecrow Press.

Darnley-Smith, R. and Patey, H. (2003) *Music Therapy.* London, Thousand Oaks, New Delhi: Sage Publications.

Hart, M. (1990) *Drumming at the Edge of Magic: A Journey into the Spirit of Percussion.* New York, NY: HarperCollins.

Jackert, L., Rio, R., Adler, R., Manthey, C., Geiger, J., Niles, S., and Schellin, K. (2003) *Music Therapy and Elderly Persons: Innovative Approaches.* American Music Therapy Association Pre-Conference Institute Publication. Silverspring, MD: AMTA.

Peters, J. S. (2000) *Music Therapy: An Introduction.* Springfield, IL: Charles C. Thomas.

Redmond, L. (1997) *When the Drummers Were Women.* New York, NY: Random House.

VanWeelden, K. and Cevasco, A. (2007) 'Repertoire recommendations by music thera-pists for geriatric clients during singing activities.' *Music Therapy Perspectives 25* (1), 4–18.

INDEX